THE AU

C000060165

Wong Kiew Kit, popularly known as S
successor of Venerable Jiang Nan from
China and Grandmaster of Shaolin Wahnam Institute of Kungfu and
Qiqong. He received the "Qiqong Master of the Year" Award during the
Second World Congress on Qiqong held in San Francisco in 1997.

He is an internationally acclaimed author of books on the Shaolin arts and
Buddhism including Introduction to Shaolin Kung Fu (1981), The Art of
Qiqong (1993), The Art of Shaolin Kung Fu (1996), The Complete Book
of Tai Chi Chuan (1996), Chi Kung for Health and Vitality (1997), The
Complete Book of Zen (1998), The Complete Book of Chinese Medicine
(2002), The Complete Book of Shaolin (2002), Sukhavati:The Western
Paradise (2002) and The Shaolin Arts (2002).

Since 1987, Sifu Wong has spent more time teaching qiqong than kungfu,
because he feels that while kungfu serves as an interesting hobby, qiqong
serves an urgent public need, particularly in overcoming degenerative and
psychiatric illnesses.

Sifu Wong is one of the few masters who have generously introduced the
once secretive Shaolin Qiqong to the public, and has helped many people
to obtain relieve or overcome so-called "incurable" diseases like
hypertension, asthma, rheumatism, arthritis, diabetes, migraine, gastritis,
gall stones, kidney failure, depression, anxiety and even cancer.

He stresses the Shaolin philosophy of sharing goodness with all humanity,
and is now dedicated to spreading the wonders and benefits of the Shaolin
arts to people all over the world irrespective of race, culture and religion.

By the same author

Complete Book of Zen
(Available in English, Spanish, Greek, Italian, Russian and Hebrew)

Art of Shaolin Kung Fu
(Available in English, Greek, Russian, Polish and Italian)

Complete Book of Tai Chi Chuan
(Available in English, Portuguese, Italian, Greek, Dutch, Russian and Spanish)

Chi Kung for Health and Vitality
(Available in English, Polish and Portuguese)

Art of Chi Kung
(Available in English, Russian, German, Spanish and Greek)

Introduction to Shaolin Kung Fu
(Available in English)

Complete Book of Chinese Medicine
(Available in English and Spanish)

Complete Book of Shaolin
(Available in English)

Sukhavati: Western Paradise
(Available in English)

Master Answers Series: The Shaolin Arts
(Available in English)

CONTENTS

EDITORIAL NOTE

Despite the wealth of information that is easily available today, many have personally written to Sifu Wong, requesting for more. Hence resulting in the publication of the **Master Answers Series.**

Since this is the first of a series of books to be published under our **Master Answers Series** , this book is designed in a way to provide prospective students, beginners, senior students and perhaps even disciples and overview of the entire story of the wonderful Shaolin Arts so that the tremendously rich history of the arts can be introduced to the current generation and at the same time maintained for the benefit of future generations.

We hope you will enjoy this book as much as we have enjoyed putting it together.

LIST OF ILLUSTRATIONS

History

Question

I know that there used to be 5 Shaolin temples in China, please correct me if I am wrong, but some of them were destroyed.

Which ones are left?

Thanx, Taiwan, Republic of China (August 1999)

Answer

There were really two Shaolin Temples, one in Henan province and the other in Fujian. Both were destroyed, but the northern temple in Henan has been restored by the Chinese government in Beijing.

The government has found the site of the southern temple and is contemplating to restore it too.

There were other temples which followed the tradition of Shaolin.

Two notable examples were the Long Tan Temple (or Dragon's Pool Temple) in Shangtung province, from where Tan Tui Kungfu developed (famous in Chinese circles, not not well known among non-Chinese), and Xi Chan Temple (or Western Zen Temple) in Guangdong, which played a crucial role in the development of many southern Shaolin styles.

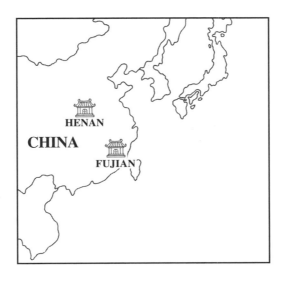

Location of The Shaolin Temples

Question

Can you tell me if it is true that the Shaolin people were attacked and killed by a Chinese Emperor who lived at the temple, learnt their secrets, betrayed them, hired the Lamas from Tibet, using a weapon translated as 'bleeding front' (a trap like thrown weapon with a rope) joined forces to destroy the Shaolin?

If this is true, how is it that the Lamas, being Buddhist, could take part in such a plot?

Mike, USA (February 2000)

Answer

Yes, it was true that the southern Shaolin Monastery at Quanzhou was razed to the ground and many of its monks and secular disciples were killed by the Qing (Manchurian) army, helped by hired Lamas from Tibet.

This expedition was ordered by the Manchurian emperor, Yong Cheng, who earlier infiltrated into the Shaolin Monastery to learn kungfu. One of the monks who escaped was the Venerable Jiang Nan, from whom my lineage derived.

Religion was never a issue in this razing of the Shaolin Monastery; it was solely political. The Shaolin Monastery had become a revolutionary center to overthrow the Manchurian government, and certainly no Manchurian emperor would tolerate this. The Lama kungfu experts came as mercenaries, not as missionaries.

The Lamas used a deadly flying weapon known as "Huit Tik Tze", which may be translated literally as "blood drops machine" or figuratively as "bleeding front". It was, as you have said, a razor-filled trap-like thrown weapon with a rope or chain which effectively decapitates an opponent's head.

Exploiting Shaolin Kungfu information provided by the emperor, the Lamas had practiced with their secret weapons to perfection before their assault.

There was also the burning of another southern Shaolin Monastery. The Venerable Chee Seen, who escaped from the southern Shaolin Monastery at Quanzhou, secretly rebuilt a smaller monastary at Jiulian Mountain.

Many southern Shaolin heroes like Hoong Hei Khoon, Fong Sai Yoke and Luk Ah Choy who later spread Shaolin Kungfu to posterity, learnt in this southern Shaolin Monastery at Juilian Mountain.

Betrayed by a disciple, Ma Ling Yi, this second southern Shaolin Monastery was also razed to the ground by the Qing army, led by the Taoist Priest Pak Mei, who was a Shaolin grandmaster and senior classmate of Chee Seen, but who sided with the Qing government.

The site of this other southern Shaolin Monastery has not yet been found.

Shaolin Tradition

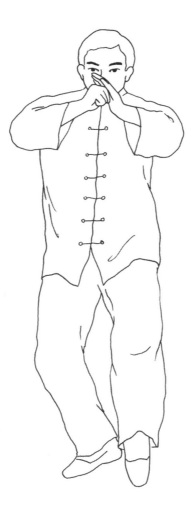

Traditional Shaolin Greeting or Salutation Pattern
known as Dragon and Tiger Appear

Addressing the Master

Question

My teacher is my Si Fu, his teacher my Si Gung. What is the appropriate title for the teacher of my Si Gung and his own teacher?

How do we address older generations? Is there any term for the founder? What is the meaning and difference between the following terms or titles: Si Tai Gung, Si Jo, Jo Si, Jung Si?

Pavel, Czech Republic (September 2000)

Answer

Your si-gung's teacher is called si-tai-gung, and his teacher is called si-jo. The founder of a system or the head of a generation line is called jo-si.

Jung-si means "teacher of the tradition". This title is usually addressed to the living head of a system. It is also sometimes addressed to a famous master.

Let us take this generation line as an example. Chee Seen —> Lok Ah Choy —> Wong Kai Ying —> Wong Fei Hoong —> Lam Sai Weng —> Lam Jo.

Lam Jo would address Lam Sai Weng as sifu, Wong Fei Hoong as si-gung, Wong Kai Ying as si-tai-gung, and Lok Ah Choy as si-jo. Anyone in this generation line from Wong Fei Hoong downward, including students today, would address Chee Seen, being the head of the generation line, as jo-si.

Technically, Lok Ah Choy and Wong Kai Ying could also address Chee Seen as jo- si, but usually they would not because they were close enough to call him si-gung and sifu respectively.

Chee Seen is the jung-si of the system. But Lok Ah Choy, Wong Kai Ying, Wong Fei Hoong and Lam Sai Weng, being famous masters, can rightly be referred to as jung-si too.

Qualities of a Good Master

Question

Ultimately, my goal is to find a good tai chi or chi kung master and I am a bit confused on how to go about it. This page helped me some to make sense out of what it is that I am looking for, and it is that spiritual or "mind" chi kung you described.

What questions should I ask a prospective teacher to help ensure my satisfaction with their interpretation of the art?

Donald, USA (May 1998)

Answer

My section on **Qualities of a Good Master** above should provide some useful information for your needs. But of course good masters are very rare nowadays.

What questions you should ask depends on numerous variables like your understanding of the art, your abilities and needs, your immediate objectives, your long-term aspirations as well as whether the teacher in question is a genuine master or a self-taught instructor who has just completed a weekend seminar on chi kung conducted by another self-taught instructor.

For example, if you, like most people in the West, regard chi kung as some form of gentle exercise that you can readily pick up from a gym or from a book, you may ask something like "How many techniques I am going to learn from you and what is your fee?"

If you regard chi kung as a rare opportunity for personal development and the teacher you are talking to is one who can make this come true, you may ask "Master, I am prepared to train hard, can you please accept me as a student and teach me according to what you think is best?"

Facing a self-taught instructor, you should politely ask questions like "Can practicing chi kung cure my backache?", "How and why chi kung can cure backache?" and "Can you please give some examples of people whose backache you have cured?"

Asking a genuine master such questions, even if you do so politely, is both unnecessary and rude.

Question

My fear and problem is how to find a proper master, how to recognize him?

I am a perfectionist and want to do little but 100% good rather then a lot and bad.

Sanjay, USA (September 1999)

Answer

Finding a real master is a big problem concerning any serious student.

The market today is littered with mediocre instructors, some of whom do not actually know what they are teaching, but finding a real master is like finding a gem. This is quite inevitable — it is a fact of life.

A lot of people would want to be masters, and some imagine themselves to be masters, but only a handful out of many thousands would actually train diligently for years to perfect their art to become masters.

The hallmark of a master is that he excels in the performance of his art.

An instructor who teaches Tai Chi but does not know any self-defense, or an instructor who teaches qigong but has never experienced any energy flow — a situation that is not uncommon nowadays — is certainly not a master; he is not even a true practitioner of his art.

But more important than asking whether your teacher is a master, is to ask yourself whether you are a deserving student.

If one is unwilling to travel some distance to his teacher, or devote some time daily for training, or address his teacher respectfully, he does not even deserve to learn the real art.

If you practice diligently, as long as what you practice is genuine stuff, you can still attain a very high level without having a master to be your teacher.

Question

Explain to me please your relation with the monk of Shaolin monastery of whom you are the successor of the 4th generation.
Roberto, Italy (April 2000)

Answer

About 150 years ago the Jing Dynasty army attacked and burned the southern Shaolin Monastery. Only top Shaolin masters escaped.

One of these was the monk Jiang Nan. He escaped to the south, with the Jing army trailing him. He had one mission in life, which was to pass on the Shaolin arts to one successor.

After about 50 years of searching, he found Yang Fatt Khun at the border between Thailand and Malaysia, Yang who was an expert at the phoenix-fist was then in his twenties. He was a traveling medicine-man who demonstrated kungfu to attract customers to his mobile roadside stall.

The Venerable Jiang Nan observed Yang's kungfu demonstration every night.

On the seventh night, after the crowd had dispersed the Venerable Jiang Nan approached Yang and told him that despite the loud applaud he had received from the crowd, his was not real kungfu but "flowery fists and embroidery kicks", a figurative term meaning that his kungfu was not effective for real fighting, and was meant only for demonstration.

Yang was surprised because he had often used his kungfu effectively to ward off Muai Thai fighters who frequently troubled him in his traveling.

The monk told him that he needed not accept the opinion but to test it in a friendly sparring. "Kungfu is meant for fighting, and not meant for demonstration", the Shaolin monk told the traveling medicine-man.

This saying has come down to our school, Shaolin Wahnam, as a basic tenet.

To his utter surprise, Yang found that this eighty-year old monk, while never hurting him, played him about like a child. Yang Fatt Khun then begged the Venerable Jiang Nan to teach him kungfu.

When Yang Fatt Khun was in his seventies he accepted a young man called Ho Fatt Nam, who was already well trained in seven styles of martial arts and who earned his living as a professional Muai Thai fighter.

At first Yang rejected Ho's persistent entreaties to be a student. When he ran out of excuses to reject Ho, Yang told Ho that he was no longer teaching kungfu (which was true if it was taken to mean teaching kungfu publicly).

One night with the help of Yang's senior student, Ho managed to "sneak" into their secret training hall and caught Yang teaching kungfu. Ho came prepared with the traditional gifts to offer a master. He prostrated before Yang and offered the gifts. Placing the gifts on the altar dedicated to past Shaolin masters, Yang remarked, "This is Heaven's will" (that I should accept him as my student).

Every year Yang Fatt Khun conducted a grand sparring competition amongst his students to choose the top ten disciples, as was the tradition in the southern Shaolin Monastery in the past.

From an unranked position, Ho Fatt Nam gradually rose over the years to the third position. In fact his name, which was given by his teacher, is an indication of his third position.

Yang Fatt Khun named his four top disciples Fatt Tung, Fatt Seai, Fatt Nam, and Fatt Pak, which means Spiritual Teaching of the East, West, South and North. When Yang Fatt Khun announced his official retirement, he named Ho Fatt Nam as his successor — as Fatt Tung was already in his eighties, and Fatt Seai had gone back to China.

Like my master himself in his own time, I was one of Sifu Ho Fatt Nam's last students.

Earlier I learnt from Sifu Lai Chin Wah, who was better known as Uncle Righteousness, and from Sifu Chee Kim Thong, respectively the patriarch of Hoong Ka Kungfu and of Wuzu Kungfu. Later I learnt from Sifu Choe Hoong Choy, the patriarch of Choe Family Wing Chun Kungfu.

It was no coincidence that I learnt from the patriarchs of the respective styles. Being an idealist, I wanted to learn from the best. Except for Uncle Righteousness from whom I learnt through sheer luck (or was it?), I spent much time and effort searching for masters.

My school, Shaolin Wahnam, was named after my two masters, Sifu Lai Chin Wah and Sifu Ho Fatt Nam, as a token of appreciation for their kindness and generosity in teaching such wonderful Shaolin arts.

Masters and Heroes from the Past

Question
The main reason I am writing to you is for my own quest for knowledge. I have done as much research as possible.

I am fascinated by the history of Chinese martial arts, particularly when it comes to famous masters, such as Yue Fei (Ngok Fei), Huo Yuan Jia (Fok Yuen Jia), Gu Ru Zhang (Ku Yu Cheung), Hung Hei Goon, and Shao Lin Hai Deng Fa Shi (Siu Lum Hoi Tung Fut Si).

Is there any information you could give me on these legendary masters?
Paul, UK (August 1999)

Answer
Yue Fei or **Ngok Fei** in Cantonese pronunciation was a famous Song Dynasty marshal, deified by later generations as a god of martial art. His martial art training was Shaolin. He was the founder or first patriarch of Hsing Yi Kungfu, Eagle Claw Kungfu and Yiejiaquan (Yue Family Kungfu).

When he was a child, his mother tattooed on his back the following Chinese words, "jing zhong bao guo", which means "extreme loyalty to repay the kingdom".

Being filial to his mother (even long after her death), Yue Fei followed his mother's tattooed words to a fault. (Anyone who thinks that being filial to one's parents is sissy should draw some inspiration from this god of martial art.)

When Yue Fei successfully prevented the Tartars at the border from invading China, the emperor instigated by a treacherous prime minister who had been bribed by the Tartars, sent out imperial decrees to recall him to the capital.

Imperial decrees were engraved in gold plates. Decrees after decrees were sent out but the gold plates were intercepted on the way by kungfu masters because they knew of an imperial plot to kill Yue Fei as soon as he arrived at the palace.

But, alas, the twelfth gold plate reached Yue Fei. He also knew he would die if he returned to the capital, and despite the army begging him not to go, he returned, for being true to his mother's words, not obeying the emperor's order would be disloyal.

True enough, when Yue Fei returned to the capital, the emperor framing a crime on him, ordered his head chopped off. Soon, without Yue Fei defending the border, the Tartars overran north China.

Huo Yuan Jia (Fok Yun Kap) was a Northern Shaolin master known for Mizongyi, or the Art of Deceptive Footwork.

He lived in the times of the early Chinese republic when China was like a piece of cake eyed by many foreign powers, and when foreigners called the Chinese the sick men of East Asia. But Huo Yuan Jia was nicknamed the Yellow-Face Tiger because of his martial art prowess.

To help his countrymen become strong and healthy, Huo Yuan Jia founded Chin Wu Athletic Association in Shanghai, which was dedicated to the spread of genuine kungfu.

Chin Wu, which literally means "Essence of Martial Art", has branches in many countries, especially in South East Asia. Huo Yuan Jia also formulated a beautiful code of philosophy to help Chin Wu members attain all-round development.

But today, and this is strictly my opinion, not many Chin Wu members could measure up to the aspirations of their great founder; much of the kungfu taught in numerous Chin Wu branches today is meant for demonstration rather than for combat, and the expression "we practice kungfu for health, not for fighting" is common among many members.

This is perhaps quite inevitable as many members of the executive committees that manage Chin Wu branches today are successful businessmen rather than kungfu masters, who while generous in their financial donation for the upkeep of the various Chin Wu branches may not be able to differentiate between demonstrative and combat kungfu.

Many Japanese martial art masters traveled to China to challenge the Chinese masters. Huo Huan Jia defeated them quite easily.

According to a popular belief, Huo Huan Jia was poisoned by his cook who had been bribed by some foreigners. He was taken to a foreign hospital in Shanghai where he soon died.

Gu Ru Zhang (Ku Yu Cheung) was another famous Northern Shaolin master who defeated many foreign martial art masters, especially from Russia and Japan. He is best known for his Iron Palm.

Anyone familiar with the western concept of muscles and strength, seeing his deceptively fragile physique could never believe how powerful Gu Ru Zhang was. He would place more than ten bricks one on top of another on the ground, without any support below.

With an apparently gentle tap on the top brick, this fragile looking Shaolin master could send his internal force down the remaining bricks and break them all! It is understandable that many modern martial artists may not believe this was possible.

Once, after seeing Gu Ru Zhang's demonstration, a skeptical spectator suspected that the bricks had been tempered with beforehand. He changed all the bricks which were to be used in another demonstration the next day.

The following day, without knowing that the bricks had been changed. Gu Ru Zhang piled the bricks up. The spectator expected Gu Ru Zhang to be put to shame. As usual the master slapped on the top brick with his palm; all the other bricks broke.

One day a stuntman from Russia brought in a trained horse and challenged the sick men of East Asia to tame it. When many Chinese were hurt by the horse, the stuntman insulted the Chinese people saying that with all their Chinese kungfu they were no better than a horse.

This angered Gu Ru Zhang.

He walked towards the horse, and gave one slap of his Iron Palm on its body. The horse collapsed and died immediately. The people, Chinese as well as foreigners, were surprised.

There was no mark of injury on the horse's body, but when they cut it open they found that many of its internal organs were smashed.

Hoong Hei Goon, which is a more popular pronunciation in Cantonese than the Mandarin pronunciation of **Hung Xi Guan**, was a great Southern Shaolin master with far-reaching influence on martial arts of the world today.

He is often described as the founder of Hoong Ka (Hung Gar) Kungfu. Actually he did not invent Hoong Ka Kungfu, he passed on to posterity what he had learnt from his master.

For a few generations after him, the style of kungfu he passed down was still called Shaolin, although the term "Hoong Ka" which means "Hoong Family" was also used. It is only in modern times that the term "Hoong Ka Kungfu" has become popular.

Hoong Hei Goon was a distinguished disciple of the Venerable Chee Seen, the abbot of the southern Shaolin Monastery in Fujian Province, and the First Patriarch of Southern Shaolin Kungfu. "Che Seen", or Zhi Zhan in Mandarin, means "Extreme Kindness".

After the burning of the monastery, Hoong Hei Goon escaped to Guangdong Province, and established a school teaching Southern Shaolin Kungfu. He married a female kungfu master called Fong Chet Leong who specialized in the Crane style. Hoong Hei Goon incorporated the Crane style of his wife into his Tiger style, resulting in the famous Tiger-Crane Set of Hoong Ka Kungfu.

Probably the most well known Hoong Ka, or Hung Gar Kungfu today, the style one frequently sees in Hong Kong movies depicting Shaolin heroes, comes from the lineage of the legendary southern Shaolin hero named Wong Fei Hoong.

It is illuminating that Wong Fei Hoong was not descended directly from Hoong Hei Goon, but from his junior classmate Lok Ah Choy.

Hai Deng Fa Shi (Hoi Theng Fatt Si) was a Northern Shaolin master of the most recent times. Because of frequent illness when he was a child, he took up Shaolin Kungfu to improve his health. Later he became a monk. His specialties include the Shaolin arts of Two-Finger Zen and Plum-Flower Formation.

For his martial art training, the Venerable Hai Deng literally stood vertically upside-down on two fingers for hours. His two fingers were so powerful that he could pierce through buffalo's hide with just one jab.

When a Japanese master mentioned that Shaolin Kungfu could no longer be found in China, the Venerable Hai Deng cme out from his self imposed retreat to demonstrate genuine Shaolin arts. He was invited to become the kungfu grandmaster at the Shaolin Monastery in Henan Province.

Perhaps due to policy differences, the Venerable Hai Deng later resigned from the monastery, where today modern wushu rather than traditional Shaolin Kungfu is taught, though not inside the monastery itself but in the numerous wushu schools around the monastery and often conducted by monastery monks.

One of Hai Deng Fa Shi's distinguished disciples is the great chi kung master, Yan Xin, considered by the present Chinese government as a national treasure.

Question

I have heard about "Ten Tigers of Shaolin Temple", layman disciples of Fujian Shaolin — Hung Heigun (Hong Xiguan), Foong Saiyuk (Fang Shiyu), Wu Waikin (Hu Huiqian) etc.

Can you briefly tell us more about these southern heroes?

Pavel, Czech Republic (November 19999)

Answer

These Southern heroes are known as the **"Ten Great Disciples of Shaolin"**, or "Sil Lam Sap Tai Tei Tze" in Cantonese or "Shao Lin Shi Da Di Zi" in Mandarin.

Different grandmasters at the Shaolin Monastery logically had different sets of ten top disciples, but the most popular in kungfu legends were the ten great disciples of the Venerable Chee Seen.

These ten great disciples of the Shaolin Monastery were not placed according to their seniority in learning from the master, but according to their performance in a grand annual free sparring competition.

This tradition was practiced in the southern Shaolin Monastery; I am not sure if it was also practiced in the northern Shaolin Monastery.

Wu Wai Thein was not one of Chee Seen's top students. In his haste to avenge his father's death, he stole out of the monastery via a ditch before he could complete his basic training. Even so, he was a good fighter, specializing in the Flower Set.

The Ten Great Disciples of Shaolin during the time Chee Seen was the abbot were as follows.

The Venerable Harng Yien was the most senior as well the foremost of Chee Seen's disciples. Unlike the others who were frequently involved in fighting, he was also the most peace-loving. He placed spiritual cultivation far above combat efficiency. Paradoxically, or perhaps because of this spiritual focus, he was also the best fighter among the ten.

The Venerable Sam Tuck was the second best. He and Harng Yien were the only two monks among the top ten disciples; the other eight were lay persons. Later Sam Tuck became the abbot of Sai Sim (or Xi Chan) Monastery in Guangdong, where many Southern Shaolin heroes gathered.

After the burning of the Shaolin Monastery, **Hoong Hei Khoon** escaped to Fatt San in Guangdong where he set up his kung fu school called Siew Lam Hoong Goon, which means the Hoong School of Shaolin Kungfu. His style of kungfu is now popularly known as Hoong Ka (Hung Gar) or Hoong Family Kungfu.

Luk Ah Choy was a Manchurian, not a Han Chinese. But, of course, although the Shaolin disciples vowed to overthrow the Manchurian government, they loved Luk Ah Choy as a brother. He was instrumental in spreading Shaolin Kungfu to posterity.

Miu Choi Fa was Miu Hein's daughter. She herself and all her three sons, How Yoke, Mei Yoke and Sai Yoke learnt from Chee Seen. She was expert in the Plum Flower Single Knife. Sadly, she was killed by a rain of arrows while defending the monastery from burning.

Thoong Chein Kern was another Manchurian. His surname was "Thoong", and "Chein Kern" which means "Thousand Pounds" in Cantonese, was his nickname because his arms and horse-stance were very powerful.

Lin Swee Hin was a son of Lin Karn Yew, a great general who helped the Manchurian government to subdue rebellions in Tibet and Mongolia. But he was later killed by the emperor who feared his extraordinary military talents. His son, Lin Swee Hin, first learnt from Fung Tou Tuck but when he found out that his teacher sided with the Qing government, he turned to Chee Seen.

Foong Sai Yoke was often known as Len Chye Yoke, or Handsome Yoke. His most celebrated occasion which also shot him to fame instantly happened when he was only about fifteen years old.

A kungfu master nicknamed Tiger Lei with his insulting slogan "Hitting all Guangdong with a fist, and striking Suzhow and Hangzhow with a kick" was unbeaten for weeks, yet was defeated by Foong Sai Yoke.

Li Choi Ping and Miu Choi Fa were the only two woman disciples of Chee Seen. Li Choi Ping was very good with the Shaolin sword.

Ma Ling Yi was the last of the ten top disciples. He was an orphan picked up by Chee Seen and brought to the monastery. Yet, he betrayed the very people who had cared for and loved him.

Shaolin Kungfu

Question

What does Shaolin Kungfu represent? What is the purpose of learning this style?

Juan, Mexico. (September 1997)

Answer

Shaolin Kungfu is the style of martial art first developed at the Shaolin Monastery in China, and is now practiced by many people in various parts of the world irrespective of race, culture and religion.

Many kungfu styles branched out from Shaolin Kungfu, and some examples include Eagle Claw Kungfu, Praying Mantis Kungfu, Hoong Ka Kungfu, Choy-Li-Fatt Kungfu and Wing Chun Kungfu.

In my opinion, which is also shared by many other people, Shaolin Kungfu represents the pinnacle of martial art development. Indeed, as early as the Tang Dynasty in China more than a thousand years ago, the saying "Shaolin Kungfu is the foremost martial art beneath heaven" was already popular.

The main purpose of learning Shaolin Kungfu is to have a complete program of personal development from the most basic to the most advanced levels. At the physical level, Shaolin Kungfu provides health, fitness, agility and vitality, besides the ability to defend ourselves. At the emotional level, Shaolin Kungfu gives us joy and tranquillity.

Shaolin Kungfu trains us to be mentally focussed, and enables us to expand our mind. At its highest level, Shaolin Kungfu leads to spiritual fulfillment, irrespective of religion. Obviously, Shaolin Kungfu is not just a fighting art.

It is also significant to note that an important aspect of the Shaolin teaching is direct experience, which in this case means that a Shaolin disciple does not merely talk about good health and mind expansion, or just read up on spirituality, but actually experience these benefits.

If he does not experience, according to his developmental stage, the appropriate results Shaolin Kungfu is purported to give, he should seriously review his training.

Different Types of Shaolin Kungfu

Question

I wish to ask you what the advantages and disadvantages of long-reaching strike used in Northern Shaolin had over the close combat of Southern Shaolin Kungfu.
Gurmeet, UK (December 1999)

Answer

Long range kungfu is good for fighting in open plains as in north China, whereas short range kungfu is good for fighting in narrow lanes as in south China.

Long range kungfu makes much use of kicking attacks, whereas short range kungfu makes much use of hand techniques, like the Eagle Claw.

Saying that Northern Shaolin is long range and Southern Shaolin short range is only speaking relatively. Both versions of Shaolin Kungfu have both long and short range. Eagle Claw Kungfu, for example, is Northern Shaolin but has many short range hand techniques.

Question

Do you know anything about two old northern Shaolin forms I found on the internet?

They are called Shaolin Bao Cuan Quan (Shaolin Running Panther Boxing) and Shaolin Bao Zi Chui (Panther Strike)?
Robert, USA (July 1999)

Answer

Yes, but I know only very little, and the very little is that many sets or forms from different styles may have these same names. Secondly, "Boxing" is an inaccurate translation of the Chinese term "Quan". A better translation is "kungfu set".

Question

I have heard of Shaolin Lohan Boxing — is this the basic Shaolin Boxing set that has to be learnt before taking the advanced forms like Five Animals?
Chi Wai, England (June 1999)

Answer

The original Shaolin Lohan Set was the prototype set of Shaolin Kungfu, from which thousands of Shaolin Kungfu sets developed over time. This prototype set was developed from the Eighteen Lohan Hands, which was taught by the great Bodhidharma between the years 527 and 536 in the northern Shaolin Monastery.

There is a style of kungfu that specializes in the Lohan Set, and this is the school of Lohan Kungfu. It is a Northern Shaolin style. The Lohan Set is also very popular among Southern Shaolin styles. Much of Hung Gar and Choy-Li-Fatt, for example, is based on the Lohan Set.

While the Lohan Set was the fountainhead of Shaolin Kungfu, one does not need to start his Shaolin training with this set. In fact the Lohan Set, of which there are now numerous versions, is an advanced set, taught only to students with many years of experience.

On the other hand, one can become a Shaolin master without even knowing the Lohan Set. Wing Chun Kungfu, for example, pays little attention to the Lohan Set. This was because the specialty of the Shaolin nun Ng Mooi, who taught kungfu to Yim Wing Chun (the founder of Wing Chun Kungfu), was the Flower Set; the Lohan Set which is favorable to those of bigger size, is generally not suitable for women. The Flower Set was developed from the prototype Five-Animal Set, with emphasis on the Snake and the Crane.

I think the word "boxing" in such terms like "Lohan Boxing" and "Shaolin Boxing", which are sometimes used in the West to refer to Lohan Kungfu and Shaolin Kungfu, is inappropriate, because it can give a false impression that Lohan Kungfu or Shaolin Kungfu is similar to western boxing.

In fact, they are vastly different. Similarly, terms like "Lohan Fist" and "Shaolin Fist" are inappropriate.

This inappropriate use of the words "boxing" and "fist" is due to an inappropriate translation from the Chinese terms "Lohanquan" and "Shaolinquan", which refer to the style of Lohan Kungfu and the style of Shaolin Kungfu. Sometimes they can also refer to a Lohan Kungfu set or a Shaolin Kungfu set.

"Quan" when referring to a kungfu style is the shortened form for "quan-fa"; and "quan" when referring to a kungfu set is the shortened form for "quan-tao" (pronounced like "ch'uan th'ao"). The "tao" in "quan-tao" is different from the "tao" in "Taoism", which is spelt as "Daoism" in romanized Chinese.

Although "quan-fa" word by word literally means "fist-technique", the compound word as a whole idiomatically means a system of martial art. Hence "Shaolinquan" or "Taijquan" is not "Shaolin fist techniques" or "Taiji fist techniques" but "Shaolin Martial Art" or "Taiji Martial Art", which includes not only fist techniques but also weapons, force training and martial art philosophy.

Question

My question relates to the various styles of southern Shaolin Kungfu.

I would appreciate any advice you have concerning my choice of style — I am attracted to the 5 animal style of Shaolin Fist, and also the Tiger/Crane style of Hung Gar Fist.

Chi Wai, England (June 1999)

Answer

Some famous styles of Southern Shaolin Kungfu are Wing Chun, Hung Gar (Hoong Ka) and Choy-Li-Fatt. The Five-Animal Set is found in both Hung Gar and Choy-Li-Fatt, whereas the Tiger-Crane Set is a famous set of Hung Gar.

Interestingly, I have learnt a Tiger-Crane Set in the Choe Family version of Wing Chun Kungfu, and this set is different from the Hung Gar Tiger-Crane Set (which I also have learnt).

If you wish to have a taste of Shaolin Kungfu in general, the Five-Animal Set is an ideal choice. You could either choose the one from Hung Gar or from Choy-Li-Fatt.

Question

My question is about the Five-Animal Set. I have only found vague references to sets and forms which are based on a specific animal of the five, such as the White Crane form.

I recollect that historically monks of Shaolin were taught perhaps one or two animal forms or sets best suited to their overall personage, and that no one monk was ever taught all five forms.

Damian, USA (November 1999)

Answer

This is not true. The Five-Animal Set was an ancient Shaolin Kungfu set complete by itself; it was not a composite set made up of patterns drawn from five different sets.

In fact the reverse process is the truth.

From the Five-Animal Set, other sets developed that specialized on only one animal, such as the White Crane Set or the Black Tiger Set.

Then a whole kungfu style was built around a specialized set, such as White Crane Kungfu, Black Tiger Kungfu, Dragon Style Kungfu, and Snake Style Kungfu. There was, however, no established Leopard Style Kungfu.

Nevertheless, one should note that it did not mean a specialized style had only patterns of that particular animal. In other words, in White Crane Kungfu, for example, there are also patterns of the dragon, snake, tiger and leopard, but crane patterns predominate.

Moreover, it is not true that a kungfu exponent who knows all the five animals is necessarily better than another who knows only one animal.

In other words, if you know the Five-Animal Set or know five different sets each of one different animal, you are not necessarily a better fighter than one who knows only any one animal set.

Indeed, again the reverse is often, but not always, the case. Students initially learn all the five animals. When they have reached a master's level, they often choose only one animal to specialize in.

Question

I was curious to know if you knew what are all the animal styles of kungfu, like horse, ox, elephant, scorpion, snow leopard, tiger, eagle, bear, etc.

Michael, USA (May 1999)

Answer

First we need to differentiate a kungfu style named after an animal, from a kungfu set or a kungfu pattern named after an animal.

In Shaolin Kungfu, for example, there are many patterns named after animals, the most well known of which are the five animals of dragon, snake, tiger, leopard and crane.

Patterns like "Hungry Tiger Catches Goat" and "Golden Leopard Watches Fire" are found in Hoong Ka Kungfu and Choy-Li-Fatt Kungfu. There are also kungfu sets named after animals, like the famous Tiger-Crane of Hoong Ka, and the Five-Animal Set of Choy-Li-Fatt.

On the other hand, there are also kungfu styles called Dragon Style Kungfu, Snake Style Kungfu, Black Tiger Kungfu, and White Crane Kungfu. All these kungfu styles named after animals are derived styles from Shaolin Kungfu.

I have not heard of a Leopard Style Kungfu, although there are many leopards patterns in various kungfu styles.

I do not know all the animal styles in kungfu. Throughout the long history of kungfu, many animal styles might have been invented and then disappeared, and there have been no authoritative records of all these styles.

In recent times, there have been styles like Dog Style Kungfu and Duck Style Kungfu. These styles, however, were unknown in the past, nor are they popular today.

Perhaps the most famous of kungfu styles named after animals is Monkey Style Kungfu. Actually there are a few different styles of Monkey Kungfu, some of which may not have the term "Monkey" in their names. Dongbiquan (Through-Arm Kungfu) and Yanqingquan (Yan Qing Kungfu) are two examples.

Other very famous styles are Praying Mantis Kungfu and Eagle Claw Kungfu. There are various sub-styles of Praying Mantis, and of Eagle Claw.

I do not know of any kungfu styles named after the horse, ox, elephant, scorpion, snow leopard and bear, although there are patterns named after them, with the exception of the snow leopard.

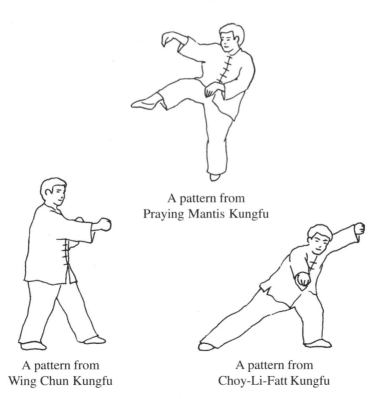

A pattern from
Praying Mantis Kungfu

A pattern from
Wing Chun Kungfu

A pattern from
Choy-Li-Fatt Kungfu

Question

I know of the 5 animal system but I have not seen anything on the 10 animal system or 12 animals.

Michael, USA (May 1999)

Answer

The five-animal system you mentioned refers to kungfu sets or kungfu patterns named after the five animals which are the dragon, snake, tiger, leopard and crane found in Shaolin Kungfu and its derivative styles like Hoong Ka and Choy-Li-Fatt.

The ten-animal system refers to a kungfu set in Hoong Ka Kungfu, purported to be invented by Wong Fei Hoong or by his disciples. Besides the five fundamental animals mentioned above, the supplementary five are lion, elephant, horse, monkey and jaguar.

The twelve animals refer to the dragon, tiger, monkey, horse, tortoise, cockerel, hawk, swallow, snake, kite, eagle and bear of Xingyiquan (Hsing Yi Kungfu).

Question

I have been instructed on the uses of Monkey's Paw and Monkey strikes, the stances and characters of the Five Monkeys and Monkey cross kicks and low stance front kicks.

Are there any techniques your are aware of that I might not know?

I understand that each character of the Five Monkeys takes on their own flavor of each technique, but I am not aware of any techniques other than those I have listed.

If you might know of any others or anyone who might, I would be grateful for that information.

Todd, USA (July 1998)

Answer

Monkey Style Kungfu is well known for its agility and deceptive nature. The knuckles, elbows, knees, shins and toes are also effectively used.

You may, for example, brush away an opponent's hand attack or leg attack with the monkey paw, then, while using the other hand as a feint move across his face, thrust your monkey paw forward with your arm moving along the opponent's arm or leg, and strike his side ribs or groin with your knuckles, simultaneously thrusting your pointed toes into his ankles.

Making faces at the opponent to cause him to loose his temper, or spitting on him to distract him are also effective monkey tactics.

Question

I was looking over your web-site and was wondering if I may ask you about the southern Chinese style of Hung Fut. I am very interested to know if this style actually exists as a recognized system.

I have never been able to find any information on Hung Fut other than it being a left handed style approximately 400 years old.

Paul, Australia (May 1999)

Answer

Hung Futt is a southern Shaolin Kungfu style based on Hung Gar Kungfu and Futt Gar Kungfu. It uses the tiger claw of Hung Gar and the Buddha Palm of Futt Gar.

This style actually exists. It is not a left handed style — it is like other styles where both hands are used, although the right hand is more often used for attack and the left for defense.

I think it developed in the later part of the Qing Dynasty in China, and therefore is only about 200 years old.

Question

Does this style originate from south China and does Hung Fut have a signature move or form, in the way that Hung Gar is well known as a tiger claw system?

How could you tell if a person knows or practices Hung Fut?

Actually, rather than ask you a lot of questions, I would be grateful if you could tell me anything you may know of this style.

Paul, Australia (May 1999)

Answer

This style originated from Guangdong Province of south China.

Its notable features are using the left hand in a Buddha Palm, and the right hand in a fist. Sometimes the tiger claws of Gung Gar are used in one or both hands. The left palm, right fist feature may reveal that the practitioner is a Hung Futt exponent, but one should also bear in mind that exponents of other styles may also use the left palm and right fist. Hung Futt exponents do not use kicks often.

Their stances are usually solid and wide, but they are also agile.

Question

I have been studying Wing Chun for about 20 months and it is quite surprising how many different styles appeared from the same set of ideas.

Jonathan, USA (May 2000)

Answer

Such developments, which were usually made in response to practical needs, enriched the repertoire of kungfu.

If we consider the fact that kungfu has a continuous history of a few thousand years and has been practiced in a region where one out of every four persons in the world lives, we can imagine how huge and rich this repertoire is, especially when compared with martial systems recently invented by a few dissatisfied martial artists and practiced by a limited number of persons.

Wing Chun Kungfu was developed by a lady kungfu master called Yim Wing Chun about 150 years ago. She practiced Shaolin Kungfu, which already had about 1500 years of history behind it.

Hence, strictly speaking, she did not invent Wing Chun Kungfu, rather she selected from what she had learnt those techniques and skills that suited her particular needs and improved them.

As a woman wearing long skirts at that time, she found wide stances and various Shaolin kicks unsuitable.

As she was relatively not as strong as male martial artists, she preferred straight attacks at opponents' vital spots, and discarded techniques like felling and locking which are more advantageous to bigger-sized persons.

Question

One thing that confuses me is the internal energy aspect. Some people say by practicing the forms you develop qi while others say that there are not any qi aspects in Wing Chun.
Jonathan, USA (May 2000)

Answer

Both statements are correct. The apparent contradiction is due to the limitation of words in expressing exactly what the speakers wanted to say, and also because their statements were made with reference to their particular situations only.

Let us take the first factor — apparent contradiction due to the limitation of words. And let us take a typical Wing Chun form — the cup fist, also called the sun-character fist as it resemblers the Chinese character for "sun"— as an example. A skillful Wing Chun exponent may perform the form as follows.

He sits at the Goat Stance. He places his left fist at his side at the level of his left breast, and his right cup fist in front of his chest. He takes a deep breath gently into his abdomen.

Then he moves his right cup fist slowly forward, simultaneously directing his qi to flow from his abdomen to his tensed right arm and generating the qi into internal force. After three repetitions, he thrusts out his cup fist fast. Here, by performing this form the exponent develops qi.

A Taijiquan exponent observing the performance may exclaim, "No, that is not qi! We may call it 'jing', but we do not call that qi." This Taijiquan exponent is quite right if we accept his concept, which is fundamental in Taijiquan, that to develop qi one has to relax totally; one cannot tense his arm.

In fact, the internal force the Wing Chun exponent will develop from that training is known as "jun jing", or Inch-Force.

Let us, for comparison, see how the Taijiquan exponent would practice his typical "peng" form to develop qi. Like the Wing Chun exponent, he takes a deep breath gently into his abdomen.

Then he moves to a right Bow-Arrow Stance and moves his right arm slowly and gently out from near his left waist to a short distance at his right eye level. Simultaneously he directs his qi to flow from his abdomen along his right arm to his right finger tips.

In his movement he is totally relaxed. If he were to tense his right arm, like what the Wing Chun exponent did, he would have stopped his qi flow. He repeats this movement a few hundred times. If he trains sufficiently he would have developed tremendous internal force, and without exerting any muscular tension could cause serious injuries with just one strike.

Now let us take the second factor — apparent contradiction due to different situations. A second Wing Chun exponent, but one who has learnt from a mediocre instructor, practices the cup fist in a similar way the first skillful Wing Chun exponent did.

But he does not pay any attention to his breathing, and does not know anything about directing qi flow. He may perform the physical form well and with much muscular strength, but if his practice is representative of what his class does, one is correct in saying there aren't any qi aspects in his Wing Chun class.

Similarly, a Taiji student, who has learnt from an instructor who teaches Taiji dance instead of genuine Taijiquan, may perform the "peng" form in a similar way the Taijiquan exponent did, but without paying attention to breathing and directing qi flow.

With sufficient training, he may be elegant and poised, as a dancer usually is, but he is unlikely to develop the kind of internal force that can fall an opponent with only one strike. One is correct in saying there aren't any qi aspects in his Taiji form practice.

Question

You stated in your web-page that kungfu without chi kung is low-level kungfu.

Does this mean that you see Wing Chun Kungfu at the same level as karate or taekwondo?

Noel, Holland (May 2000)

Answer

There is chi kung in Wing Chun too.

The two most famous chi kung manifestations in Wing Chun are "Sticking Hands" and "Inch-Force". An expert in "Sticking Hands", even when blind-folded, can sense an opponent's movements and emotions.

An expert in "Inch-Force" can cause serious damage to his opponent from a very close distance. The celebrated Bruce Lee often demonstrated his "Inch-Force" in his famous "inch-punch". To me, Wing Chun Kungfu is far above karate and taekwondo.

But the way some people practice Wing Chun is like practicing karate or taekwondo. It suggests to me that their teacher knows external Wing Chun forms but does not know its internal dimensions and its traditional methods of combat training.

Hence he has incorporated karate and taekwondo methods into his external Wing Chun forms. This is typical of many modern kungfu instructors.

Question

I love martial arts, and in the past two years I have studied Bruce Lee's Jeet Koon Do, and Wing Chun.

John, USA (December 1999)

Answer

Jeet Koon Do and Wing Chun are very effective martial arts. If your main purpose is combat efficiency, they are excellent choices.

But if you are looking for other dimensions like internal force training and spiritual cultivation, you may find arts like Shaolin and Taijiquan give you more room for expansion.

This, of course, is strictly my opinion. Many other experts, especially Jeet Koon Do and Wing Chun masters, will have different opinions, and you should also listen to their views.

Moreover, my opinion above is given relatively. If we compare a Wing Chun exponent who has trained "inch-force" with a Shaolin or Taijiquan exponent who only performs external forms, the Wing Chun exponent has much more internal force.

Question

In your work you mention that Wuzu Kungfu goes back to the Yuan Dynasty. This peaks my interest because you seem to be the only one that has information that goes back so far.

I write to ask you for information on the style's history that you did not put in your book. Anything will be greatly appreciated.

Eduardo, USA (February 1999)

Answer

Wuzu Kungfu, or Five-Ancestor Kungfu, was invented by the great Shaolin master, Bai Yi Feng, during the Yuan Dynasty by combining the five Shaolin styles of White Crane, Bodhidharma Kungfu, Lohan Kungfu, First Emperor Kungfu and Monkey Style Kungfu.

Later during the Qing Dynasty, Cai Yi Ming popularized it in the province of Fujian in south China. Hence, Wuzu Kungfu is commonly called Goh Chor Kungfu, which is the Fujian pronunciation.

In Fujian, Wuzu Kungfu was also known as Goh Chor Hok Yeong Khoon, which means Five-Ancestor "Yang" Crane Kungfu, because amongst the five composite styles, the "hard" features of the crane was the most emphasized.

It was also known as Gaik Beng Khoon, named after Cai Yi Ming — "Gaik Beng" being the Fujian dialect of "Yi Ming" which is the official Chinese pronunciation.

The Fujian master, Sifu Chee Kim Thong, from whom I learnt Wuzu Kungfu in my young days, brought Wuzu Kungfu from China to Malaysia, from where it spread to various countries, including in Europe, Australia and America. Sifu Chee first learnt kungfu from her grandmother, then from Du Yi Chuan, Lin Xian and finally from the famous lady Wuzu master Lin Yi Liang. Sifu Chee's disciple, Chan Si Ming, won the sparing championship in the first South East Asian competition.

Question

I continued my training in Tsoi Li Hoi Kungfu, or Kungfu San Soo as it is called here.

Are there any information, leads and advice you can give me in finding out more?

Ron, USA (November 1997)

Answer

"Tsoi" stands for Choy Ka Kungfu, "Li" on the other hand stands for Li Ka Kungfu, "Hoi", I think, should be "Hor" instead, as indicated in the Chinese character you provided, and was the surname of a famous southern Shaolin master who had much influence over Fatt Ka Kungfu.

Choy refers to Choy Pak Tat, the first patriarch of Choy Ka Kungfu, which is famous for its kicking techniques. Two such deadly kicks are the "organ-seeking kick", which is a snap-kick to the opponent's sex organ, and the "whirlwind kick", which uses the shin to strike at the opponent's ribs.

Li refers to Li You San, the first patriarch of Li Ka Kungfu, well known for its phoenix-eye punch. Li You San was a disciple of Pak Mei, a Taoist priest and one of the five grandmasters of Southern Shaolin.

The phoenix-eye punch, specially used to strike an opponent's vital points, is not commonly found in today's Choy-Li-Fatt Kungfu.

It is possible that this phoenix-eye punch, which demands a very high level of kungfu skill, gradually evolved to the leopard punch, which is popular in Choy-Li-Fatt Kungfu and which is more suited to en mass fighting used by Choy-Li-Fatt patriots during the Boxers' Rebellion.

"San Soo" is probably a pronunciation variation of "san sau". San Sau literally means "Miscellaneous Hands", which is a figurative way of referring to specific techniques to meet particular combat situations.

The traditional approach to sparring in kungfu training was first learning a complete kungfu set, then applying patterns of the set for combat. Choy-Li-Fatt patriots in the midst of their revolutionary work, sought a short cut to kungfu sparring.

They did away with long kungfu sets, and trained only individual techniques to meet combat situations. These individual techniques are called "san sau".

Question

I began Hung Gar Kungfu about a year ago. It was my first experience in martial arts and it has been one of the most exciting and enlightening experiences of my life so far. The lineage of our *kwoon* is directly through Wong Fei Hung. Then I moved to another place and learnt in another Hung Gar school.

To my surprise, my second sifu told me that he did not consider what I earlier learnt as real Hung Gar.

When I talked about this with my first sifu he told me he did not believe that the Hung Gar taught in the second school was real Hung Gar but some other southern style very close to Hung Gar.

At first I was surprised that two sifus of Hung Gar would not agree on their style. Then I searched on the Internet for information and learnt that Wong Fei Hung's Hung Gar is considered orthodox and other lineages of Hung Gar may differ.

I assumed that my second *kwoon* was from a different lineage and that was the source of the misunderstanding.

What should I look for that will tell me if I am practicing Hung Gar? For example, in my first *kwoon* we used to condition our fists on sandbags and our forearms on wooden posts or with training partners. Advanced students conditioned their snake fist in bowls full of gravel.

When I talked about this with students from my second *kwoon* they looked at me as if I was talking gibberish. They told me that these were not necessary and they were only for showing off.

Can this possibly be true?

Dube, Canada (January 2001)

Answer

Your situation concerns many people interested in the authenticity of their style or lineage. There are three useful guidelines to help us determine authenticity

1. lineage
2. philosophy
3. instructional material.

If you can trace your lineage directly to Wong Fei Hung, and as Wong Fei Hung is publicly acknowledged as a great Hung Gar master, then you can reasonably say ours is genuine Hung Gar.

Secondly we can examine the philosophy of the school. Hung Gar, as the direct successor of southern Shaolin, believes in both internal and external force training, but the approach is from hard to soft.

If a particular school teaches only hard, external training, like punching sandbags and striking poles, but no soft, internal training even at its advanced level, like breath control and channeling energy, one may suspect whether it is genuine Hung Gar.

The third guideline is to examine its instructional material. Hung Gar's three traditional kungfu sets are "Taming the Tiger", "Tiger and Crane" and "Iron Wire", and its famous arts are "tiger claws" and "no-shadow kicks".

If students of the school use kickboxing techniques in sparring and bounces about like Western boxers, but know little about tiger claws and no-shadow kicks, we can suspect whether the school is genuine Hung Gar.

There may, however, be complications regarding these three guideline. For example, someone might have learnt from a genuine Hung Gar master, but his training under the master was short and much of his kungfu was derived from other sources. It then becomes questionable whether he can be accepted in the Hung Gar lineage.

Or, he might have trained from a genuine Hung Gar lineage, but for some reasons this lineage transmits only elementary Hung Gar skills and techniques. Practitioners from this lineage, for example, only punch sandbags and strike poles, but know little about internal force. It would be difficult to say whether theirs is genuine Hung Gar. Normally one would say theirs is from the Hung Gar lineage but has lost Hung Gar's essence.

The three fundamental sets mentioned above are from the Wong Fei Hung's lineage. But practitioners from other genuine Hung Gar lineage may not practice these sets.

In my young days I knew of a genuine Hung Gar school that did not have any one of these sets in their repertoire. They had sets like "Cross-Roads", "Four Gates" and "Tiger Claws".

But their skills and techniques are typically Hung Gar. On the other hand, merely knowing the three fundamental sets is no guarantee that the practitioner practices genuine Hung Gar.

There are also some interesting questions regarding what is genuine Hung Gar.

If we take the definition commonly adopted by many people, but often without knowing deeply, that Hung Gar Kungfu is the style derived from Hung Hei Khoon, then Wong Fei Hung's kungfu is not Hung Gar!

Wong Fei Hung's lineage leads to Lok Ah Choy, and not to Hung Hei Khoon. There was actually no direct connection from Hung Hei Khoon to Wong Fei Hung.

The indirect connection was that Lok Ah Choy was Hung Hei Khoon's junior classmate under the Venerable Chee Seen at the southern Shaolin Temple.

In fact, Wong Fei Hung never called his kungfu Hung Gar; he called it Shaolin. His successor, Lam Sai Weng who passed on the three fundamental sets in three classics, also called his kungfu Shaolin. The term "Hung Gar" never occurred in any one of these classics. It was much later that their succeeding practitioners call their art Hung Gar.

Question
I am studying Shaolin Lau Gar Kungfu but cannot find any information anywhere.

Can you give me any help? I train in the south of England and it has become a huge part of my life.
Ben, England (April 1998)

Answer
Lau Gar Kungfu was founded by Lau Sam Ngian, a Southern Shaolin master who lived in the later part of the Qing (Ching) Dynasty in China. Lau Gar and Lau Sam Ngian are the Cantonese pronunciation. In Mandarin they are pronounced as Liu Jia and Liu San Yan.

Lau Gar means Lau's Family; it was common to name the style of kungfu after the master's surname so as to avoid using the term Shaolin because the Qing army was after Shaolin disciples.

Lau Sam Ngian was actually the master's nickname, and it means Lau Three Eyes, because there was a mark on the master's forehead that resembled a third eye. He was famous for his Shaolin staff techniques.

Information on Lau Gar Kungfu is scarce. I made a passing reference to Lau Gar Kungfu in my books, "Introduction to Shaolin Kungfu" and "The Art of Shaolin Kungfu".

Question
How many styles of Drunken Kungfu are there?
Law, Malaysia (August 2000)

Answer
There are many types of Drunken Kungfu, but the exact number is not known.

Many styles or schools of kungfu have their own forms of Drunken Kungfu, such as Drunken Praying Mantis, Drunken Lohan and Drunken Monkey. There are also Drunken Sword forms and Drunken Staff forms.

There are, however, no Drunken Kungfu forms in the internal arts of Taijiquan, Baguazhang and Xingyiquan. Drunken Kungfu also does not exist as a style or school by itself, such as in the same hierarchy as Wing Chun Kungfu, Praying Mantis Kungfu or Taijiquan.

Question

Do you know where the form "Eight Drunken Immortals" came from, and who created it? I was told all other drunken forms are derived from this form.

Is that true? Any info would be appreciated.

Law, Malaysia (August 2000)

Answer

There are also many forms of "Eight Drunken Immortals" belonging to different styles or schools of kungfu. For example, "Eight Drunken Immortals" is an important set in many Choy-Li-Fatt schools, and in Choe Family Wing Chun. The prototype of "Eight Drunken Immortals" is reputed to be from Taoist Kungfu.

As there are different sets of "Eight Drunken Immortals", there is no one inventor. These different sets were invented or developed by different masters of different kungfu styles, drawing inspiration from the prototypical "Eight Drunken Immortals" of Taoist Kungfu. I do not know who invented this prototypical set.

While the prototypical "Eight Drunken Immortals" has inspired many forms of Drunken Kungfu, it is not true that all Drunken Kungfu forms were derived from it. Drunken Monkey and Drunken Praying Mantis, two of the more famous Drunken Kungfu forms, imitate movements of the monkey and the praying mantis, although they may draw inspiration from the philosophy and techniques of the Eight Drunken Immortals.

Moreover, some Drunken Kungfu forms were derived from movements of drunken mortals, rather than from the Immortals.

Combat

Question

I saw at an international competition participants of various styles fight like children. Can kungfu really be used for fighting?

JF, Malaysia (September 1997)

Answer

Your question touches on the essence of kungfu. Yes, there is no doubt that kungfu, if practiced correctly, can be used for fighting. Kungfu that cannot be used for fighting is no longer kungfu; at best it is merely a demonstrative kungfu form.

Nevertheless, today an overwhelming majority of those who say they practice kungfu, in both the East and the West, either fight like children or use karate, taekwondo or kickboxing techniques to fight, but not the kungfu techniques that they may perform beautifully in solo practice. (Please note the point here is not their fighting ability, or whether kungfu is better or worse than other fighting arts, but whether kungfu students use kungfu to fight.)

The reason is simply that, in my opinion, they have never learnt kungfu as a martial art as it was traditionally practiced in the past. If you merely learn kungfu form, but have never learnt how to develop force and how to spar, you simply have no force and cannot spar no matter how long you might have trained in kungfu form.

Force training and sparring practice have to be approached methodologically and systematically. Skipping over a rope and lifting weights, prancing about and donning boxing groves are not traditional Shaolin ways to develop force and train sparring.

It is only sensible that if one wishes to fight like what a Shaolin exponent would do in the past, he or she must train the way a traditional Shaolin disciple did. But for various reasons, many people lack the knowledge or the patience to do so.

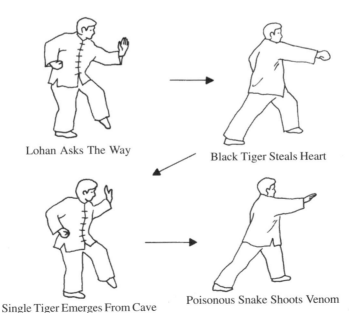

Lohan Asks The Way

Black Tiger Steals Heart

Single Tiger Emerges From Cave

Poisonous Snake Shoots Venom

Combat Sequence

Question

There is something which has bothered me for quite some time. I have observed various types of martial arts. Some include ninjado, northern Shaolin boxing, taekwondo and nam wah pai. They seem to lack a certain amount of "essence". Please allow me to explain what I mean.

The various martial arts have excellent techniques and if executed properly, could attack with deadly force. They also help a person keep fit and rank among the most physically demanding sports.

However, all these arts failed a 7th dan taekwondo instructor when he needed it most. He was brutally attacked and killed when he was caught in the middle of a gang fight, and he was only a passer-by.

This incident shook my confidence of martial arts. A person who has practiced martial arts for more than twenty years cannot even defend himself against a few men with machetes and broken bottles.

What is the use of practicing martial arts then? Where are the really useful moves when you need them? Where is the true essence of the martial arts we practice?

I understand that you, Grandmaster Wong, have performed incredible feats, as described in your web-page and books. I cannot but wonder how the most skilled person in Singapore would fare against you. I believe he would not even and remotely close to you.

Grandmaster Wong, my heart is heavy and my soul is weary. I find it hard to go on in the realm of martial arts.

Please advise me as I need help.

Lee, Singapore

Answer

Thanks for your e-mail and the kind words you said about me.

The so-called incredible feats I performed can actually be performed by anybody if he knows the training procedure and is prepared to train hard for them.

Moreover, although I strongly believe that all those who practice a martial art, any martial art including taijiquan, should be able to defend themselves, I am not a formidable fighter, and I have never aimed to be one.

What I really consider incredible about my training is that it has given me good health, much vitality, mental freshness and spiritual joy. For example, I cannot remember when I was last sick, and I could work energetically from 7.00 a.m. till 12.00 midnight without fatigue.

What I am really proud is that I have helped many people to share such benefits, including helping many people to be relieved of so-called incurable diseases like asthma, diabetes, heart problems and even cancer.

Your remark really touches on the essence of martial arts. For more than 20 years I have been concerned about the inability of most (so-called) kungfu exponents to fight. I do not demand that they must fight well, but the least is that as they learn kungfu, a martial art, they must be able to put up some form of defense even if they lose badly in a fight.

The fact is that most kungfu exponents cannot put up any semblance of defense at all, although they may perform their kungfu patterns or sets beautifully in solo demonstrations or arranged sparring.

Nevertheless, this is a very delicate and sensitive issue. While I feel strongly about it, I have to be extremely careful in my expression because not only I do not want to have kungfu people continuously coming to challenge me to test if I can fight, I do not want to hurt the feelings of kungfu "masters" (many of whom are my friends) whom I know cannot fight.

I wonder whether you have seen any kungfu sparring competitions? They were shameful. Many competitors fought like children; those who could put up some decent fighting, fought with karate, taekwondo or kickboxing techniques.

It was more shameful when "masters" employed taekwondo exponents, put on kungfu uniforms and won, and the "masters" claimed them as their own kungfu students.

In taijiquan push-hand competitions, although virtually every taijiquan master and instructor says that taijiquan does not use brute force, virtually every taijiquan competitor uses brute force, and clumsily.

The use of weight divisions in kungfu (and taijiquan) competitions is a tacit admission that weight, size and brute force count. The introduction of wushu, the modern form of demonstrative kungfu popularized by present-day China, quickens the transformation of kungfu from a martial art to a dance.

The undeniable fact is that kungfu, including taijiquan, is a martial art, and a very effective one too — if it is practiced as kungfu, and not as kung fu dance. Karate, taekwondo, aikido, judo, boxing and wrestling exponents would be no match against a genuine kungfu exponent.

A kungfu exponent would find a Siamese boxer formidable, but if he is prepared to train hard he could beat the latter too.

I must categorically clarify that this statement is not meant to belittle the other arts. In many ways, although I personally do not encourage my children and those who seek my advice to train in these arts, I generally have more respect for exponents of these arts than for those who learnt kungfu.

There are a few reasons. For example, these other exponents are true to what they seek, they can defend themselves with their arts, and they are prepared to undergo tough training, whereas those from kungfu schools do not know what they are doing or are deceiving themselves and others.

For a long time I have wanted to train a team of genuine kungfu fighters who can show the world that kungfu can be used for fighting. It does not matter if they lose so long as they use kungfu skills and techniques, and fight honorably.

But for various reasons I still have not been able to do so. It is not easy to gather a group of young men (or women) ready to train hard everyday for three years. Secondly, this project will involve heavy cost.

But probably the most important reason is my scale of priority. Personally, although I have strong sentiments over it, I do not believe that nowadays combat efficiency takes top priority in kungfu training. I do not want to subject my students to training hard for something I do not give top value for.

I always want my students to get the best, and the best is good health, vitality, mental freshness, spiritual joy irrespective of religion, and a zest for living.

Moreover, I feel the time for me to train a fighting group would be better spent to help patients cured of cancer and heart problems. It is sad that the taekwondo master you mentioned was brutally killed.

It is not easy to fight against a group of armed attackers, but I agree with you that a martial art master who has trained for 20 years should be able to come out alive when attacked by a few armed attackers.

Perhaps his death had something to do with his martial art philosophy. Korean and Japanese martial artists generally believe that it is an honor to fight, even to death. If a Japanese master were sparred his life by his attackers, he might even kill himself, not just to escape the shame of defeat but to die in honor for his art.

Chinese martial art philosophy is different. There is nothing honorable about killing oneself or being killed by others. If you cannot fight for your life, you have to run for it. It is not just an honor, but a joy to be alive.

This difference in philosophy can be traced to their different histories. Japanese martial arts were developed by samurais, who were actually cold-blooded assassins, ready to kill or die for their lords.

Korean martial arts were developed at a time when the country was oppressed by Japanese colonialists, and Korean masters were ready to die fighting the oppressors.

In contrast, Shaolin Kungfu were developed by Buddhist monks whose hallmark was compassion, and taijiquan by Taoist priests whose preoccupation was immortality. Both Shaolin and taijiquan masters loved life, their own as well as others'.

I wish to share another secret with you. My master Sifu Ho Fatt Nam, who has dedicated his life to helping others, was once attacked by more than 30 armed attackers whose objective was to kill him and his family for reasons I would not disclose here.

He fought them off. My master could have killed their leader and some other assassins (which was actually easier and safer than fighting on) but he let them go. This incident, which happened before I met my master, has great significance for me.

It confirmed not only that kungfu can be used for fighting, but that Shaolin masters are compassionate, even at times when doing so might risk their own lives.

Strictly speaking, and in my opinion, taekwondo, judo, aikido, karate, boxing and wrestling are martial sports, not martial arts.

From the perspective of Shaolin Kungfu, no experienced fighters who have survived numerous fights, would fight the way exponents of these sports would typically do.

Kicking high, for example, not only exposes your vital organs, it is technically inferior. For instance, high kicks distort good balance and minimize the effective use of other striking parts like the other leg, the two hands, shoulders, hips, etc.

If you have seen a judo match, you would have noticed how long it takes, even for a judo expert, to throw his opponent. If the opponent just jabs two fingers into the expert's eyes, or, less brutally, kicks hard at his shin, he would have foiled the expert's throw.

But of course for those who are untrained, or who are trained in kungfu dance, such kicks and throws as well as martial techniques of the other sports would be formidable.

Yet, while genuine kungfu is very effective for fighting, combat efficiency is not its best benefits. We should of course be able to defend ourselves, but if we place undue emphasis on fighting, it would distract us from other more noble aims.

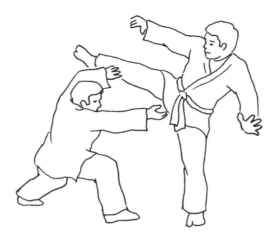

A Shaolin Kungfu technique to counter-attack
a Taekwondo high-kick

Long Lost Skills or Simply Myths

Phil Ventura, University Lecturer

At the beginning of this year I wrote to Sifu regarding studying with him in Malaysia for a month. He replied that a month's time was not necessary and that it would be more beneficial for me to spend two weeks training with him.

Given the fact that I had only been studying kungfu for around 8 months, I was doubtful about how much could be accomplished in two weeks.

Still, I had read all of Sifu's books and his web-pages and hoped that the "myths" of kungfu he writes of could be experienced. The price of the course along with airfare did seem prohibitive and I had never been out of the country but the opportunity to experience real kungfu would be worth it.

I consider myself a skeptic. I had read numerous accounts of "internal force," *qi*, and miraculous feats of strength and healing, but I was convinced these were long lost skills or simply myths.

During my first session with Sifu I was able to experience qi flow. I felt it moving through my body and was amazed to have it cause me to sway about gently. Especially since I had previously tried to practice the exercises described by Sifu in his books on qigong, but the effect was nowhere near what I felt that day.

I am convinced that one of the factors was having Sifu there to guide me and to answer my questions which put my anxieties about whether I was performing the exercises correctly to rest. As time progressed I found my experiences of qi only grew stronger.

During my training I found that even the mundane became profound. Like many other modern kungfu students, I had spent a great deal of time performing and learning sets.

After teaching me the basic patterns Sifu then led me to compose various sets of my own. But additionally, he showed me how to use the forms to practice energy management and breath control among other things.

I was amazed to find that after performing my sets numerous times, even in Malaysia's tropical climate to which I was unaccustomed, I was not tired.

In fact I felt quite refreshed and even more energetic! Subsequently, during my own practice sessions, I have found that performing my kungfu sets serves as an effective method for evoking chi flow.

All the "magical" aspects of kungfu practice did not overshadow its primary purpose, combat efficiency. Sifu taught me systematic training methods through the use of combat sequences that a kungfu student should use to train for free sparring, and ultimately combat.

Each sequence added higher levels of complexity and further tactics and strategies. They allowed me to focus on balance, timing and spacing, but also to more fully appreciate the significance of each of the patterns I had learnt.

Indeed I had read Sifu's descriptions in his book, and given my past experience tried to practice them on my own. But it was not until I studied with him that I was able to really experience the effectiveness, and elegance of each movement.

The effects of all my practice continue on. After returning home even my wife had commented on how much happier I seemed. She noted that I was much calmer and more patient, and exuded confidence.

I, too, have noticed these changes over the past few weeks. Things that previously would have caused anxiety, do not, or when they do, my mind does not abide there. In fact, I will soon be discontinuing the use of my medication for depression.

I cannot express my gratitude to Sifu for so generously sharing his Shaolin teachings with me. Nor can I ever repay him for the precious gems of Shaolin Kungfu, qigong and Zen that he has given me. I am deeply honored to call him my teacher.

Even if I never train with Sifu again, my life has been enriched immeasurably. I will continue to practice diligently what he has taught me, and hope that I will train with him further in the future.

Phil Ventura
17th September 1999
New York State, United States of America

Training

Question

How does one develop combat skills such as self-reflection, speed, timing, power, eye movement and listening to sounds?
Hendry, Indonesia (April 2000)

Answer

There are different and varied techniques to achieve these skills. But the crucial point is that one must acquire the skills from a master who has the skills, and not just learn the techniques from someone who knows the techniques.

It is difficult for the uninitiated to appreciate this point even though they may believe its verity. In other words even if I explain in detail some techniques to acquire a particular skill, someone following my explanation exactly on his own and without my personal guidance may still not acquire the skill.

But for the sake of information, I shall briefly mention some common techniques or methods used in my kungfu school to acquire the following skills.

Self-reflection is efficiently accomplished by going over selected responses to opponent's movements thousands of times. Speed is accomplished by regulating our breathing in set practice.

Timing is achieved through arranged sparring, power through stance training, and eye movement through "One Finger Shooting Zen". Listening to sound is not emphasized in my school, but can be achieved through meditation.

This division into separate, individual skills is arbitrary; in reality the skills are achieved collectively. For example, when we go over certain movements thousands of times, we accomplish not only self-reflection but also other combat skills like power, speed and timing.

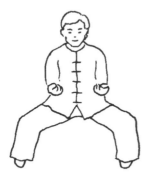

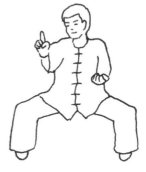

Horse-Riding Stance   One-Finger Shooting Zen

Question

How does isometric exercise differ from weight resistance exercise in terms of organ stress and the build-up of toxic waste?

Are isometric exercise sets such as the Hung-style "No Lick Kuen" less harmful than lifting weights? How?

Joshua, USA (December 1999)

Answer

I do not know enough of how isometric exercise works to comment on it competently. Genuine Hung Gar force training, like the Iron Wire Set, may look like isometric exercise but it is not. In Hung Gar force training, mind and intrinsic energy are involved, whereas in isometric exercise it is mainly physical.

It is the failure to realize the great difference between mind and energy training on one hand, and physical training on the other that many people think they can learn Hung Gar force training like the Iron Wire Set from a book or video and then having learnt the external form teach it to others.

In Hung Gar force training, if it is done correctly, you strengthen your organs and disposes off toxic waste, whereas in physical exercise like weight-lifting you stress your organs and produce toxic waste. But if you perform the force training incorrectly, you harm yourself more than in weight-lifting.

I do not know "No Lick Kuen". Perhaps it has been transcribed from Chinese into English spelling differently, or perhaps it is a new set invented by a master.

Question

How about practicing kicks versus running. I feel similarly exhausted after kick practice and running. I assume that I am practicing the kicks incorrectly.

I understood that kungfu exercises were to leave one refreshed afterwards.

Joshua, USA (December 1999)

Answer

Irrespective of whether kicking or running, if you perform them as mere physical exercise you stress your muscles and produce toxic waste.

If you incorporate chi kung into your kicking or running, you will not only have a better supply of energy for the task, you will also be more effective in toxic waste disposal.

Hence, in my kungfu school, after kicking my students will go into a spontaneous energy flow exercise.

Question

Is there a manner to reduce the harmful effects of western training, outside of your personally-guided training?

Stretching, breathing, improper practice of your chi kung (outlined in your books)?

Joshua, USA (December 1999)

Answer

A good piece of advice passed down to us by past masters is as follows. Practice regularly and progress gradually. As far as possible be natural and gentle in your training.

Even if you do not know chi kung, if you follow the above advice while performing western training methods, you can minimize much health hazard and possible serious injury, and in the end probably get better results.

Many people used to western concepts of strength and fitness may find the above advice, especially the second part, odd. How, they ask, can you be powerful when you are gentle? Consequently they put stress on their body which is not ready for the extra burden, and in their haste to get quick result they stretch themselves to their limits.

The cerebrated Bruce Lee made this serious mistake, and he paid heavily for it, dying relatively young.

Question

How should I map out my kungfu training?

Trystan, UK (August 1999)

Answer

Use the following principles to map out your training:

1. Train in all the four dimensions of kungfu, namely form, force, application and philosophy. If you just practice form, you are likely to make kungfu into gymnastics or dance.
2. Kungfu forms are means; they are not ends by themselves. You train kungfu forms so that they can be effectively used for combat and for promoting your health and vitality.

In other words, if you have been practicing kung fu forms for a year, but cannot apply them to defend yourself against even simple punches and kicks, or you still have health problems like asthma or allergies, or still feel fatigue easily and often depressed, you have wasted your time.

3. The focus of kungfu is training "kung" (spelt as "gong" in Romanized Chinese), and not on learning new techniques. A characteristic feature of "kung" training is repeatedly practice the same technique, such as hitting your palm on a bean-bag in Iron Palm training, or remaining in the same stance for 15 minutes in zhan zhuang training, every day for at least a few months.

A common feature of kungfu gymnastics or dance is learning new forms regularly and ensuring the forms are beautiful to watch.

Question

I live in a place where there are no kungfu schools and no private teachers, so I try my best on my own. I work out but I feel that something is missing in my workouts.

There are 4 parts in my complete workout: A. Power and Strength B. Flexibility C. Techniques D. Chi Kung
Igal, USA (November 1999)

Answer

It is obvious that you are dedicated to your art and is trying to make the best of what you can. Your classification of your training into the above four groups shows you have done some reading as well as thinking.

But — and this may come as a big surprise to you and many people who may think what you have done is very sensible — you have wasted your time! It is people like you, who are dedicated but are wasting their time, that I would like to help.

The problem is not with what you train, but with how you train. In fact, your classification above is a good move, but your questions and the description of your workout indicated that you have not been training correctly. You will understand more as you read on.

You may find my comments unpleasant, but they are meant to help you.

Question

Could you tell me how much time I should spare for each one of them. Workout like that will take about 2-4 hours. Each day I exercise for 1-1.5 hours.

By that time I only work on power exercises and a little of techniques.

Igal, USA (November 1999)

Answer

What you have described is typical of someone imposing western concepts on kungfu or chi kung training. This is understandable for someone from a western society and has no access to a master or a good school, and therefore has to learn from books or videos.

In such a case, he needs at least 4 hours a day, and after training daily for 20 years (or for his whole lifetime) he achieves little in terms of kungfu or chi kung. He could not, for example, defend himself or generate an internal energy flow, which are basic objectives in kungfu and chi kung training. Worse still, after all these years of training, he may not even be healthy.

You probably belong to such a case; that is why I said you had wasted your time.

Someone who has access to a mediocre school or instructor would need about 2 hours a day, but in terms of health and vitality he would achieve in 10 years what the first person above would take 20 years to achieve.

In terms of kungfu, he would still not be able to defend himself well because combat application has not been part of the training.

Someone who learns personally from a master will take far less time to achieve the same or better results.

For example, instead of spending half an hour or an hour for one exercise in each of the above four categories, students in my intensive chi kung courses need to spend only 15 minutes for just one exercise, yet they obtain benefits in all the four categories of power and strength, flexibility, techniques and chi kung!

More significantly, the result is far superior; they will achieve in 6 months what the others may not attain in 20 years, or actually in their whole lifetime. Although it may not be obvious, the reason is simple.

My students do chi kung, but the others do not; and because they do not practice chi kung, no matter for how long they train, they will not get the benefits of chi kung.

Although you, like many other people, may learn chi kung techniques from my books and practice them diligently, you are not doing chi kung although you may think you are.

As I have not seen you practice, how would I know that you have not been practicing chi kung? From your questions. If you had practiced chi kung and enjoyed its benefits, you would not have asked me the questions you asked. You would have got the answers from your own experience.

But my chi kung students would not know how to defend themselves because self defense is not an objective of the course. If they want self defense, they have to take my intensive kungfu course, where combat application and internal force training are important components.

For how long a kungfu student needs to train before he is combat efficient, depends on what and how he trains.

If he just learns from a book or a video (apart from those who are already well trained, where the book or video is only a supplement), he is unlikely to be combat efficient even if he trains for a whole lifetime.

If he learns from a good master, he should be able to handle a black-belt within three years.

Question

Anyway now I will tell you my weekly workout.

Wake up

    1.The pose of the horse rider.

    2.A little flexibility exercises.

    3.Eight Standing Pieces of Brocade.

Evening

    1.Power exercises

    2.Three sets of "Thirty Punches" with dumbbells.

    3.Sparring with dumbbells in hands

    4.Standing on hands trying to walk for 30 seconds

    5.Hitting each leg 36 times as in Thai Boxing.

Before sleep

    1.Flexibility exercises.

    2.Horse-Riding Stance.

    3.Breathing exercises.

    4.Eight Sitting Pieces of Brocade.

    5.Muscle/Tendon Changing Chi Kung (from Dr. Yang Jwing-Ming's "Muscle/Tendon Changing and Marrow /Brain Washing Chi Kung).

Igal, USA (November 1999)

Answer

You will need at least 3 hours a day to complete this routine, and by the time you have completed it you would no longer have time or energy to do other things. If you continue like this for three years you would become a wretch.

For those looking for secrets of the masters, here is one, though many people may not believe in it. Choose just one suitable force training exercise, and stick to it for at least a year.

In fact, any master seeing your routine will easily conclude that you have not really understood what kungfu or chi kung is about. You will have a better idea of your situation if you ask yourself these two questions and sincerely answer them.

What do I really want to achieve in my kungfu or chi kung training? Am I, after training in these exercises any nearer to my goals?

Question

All that I wrote I do every day, but still I feel that it is not all. Maybe power exercises should be done less or should I make any other changes? I feel that all my workouts does not worth a thing because I do not feel any progress.

I am thinking about buying a Wing Chun Dummy. Maybe then I will progress.

Igal, USA (November 1999)

Answer

You have wasted your time, and now you want to waste your money.

What are you going to do with a Wing Chun Dummy? It may be useful to those practicing Wing Chun Kungfu, but not for you.

Masters have warned that internal force training, which is what some of the exercises you mentioned aim to develop, needs to be practiced under a master's supervision, yet you are training at the same time in three or four different types of internal force on your own when you do not have even elementary kungfu experience.

On the other hand, masters have advised that to get the best result, and in the most economical time, learn from a master, yet you are trying different things on your own, presumably from books. If you are serious about kungfu or chi kung, search for a master.

This, of course, is not easy. If there were a master in your area dying to teach you, you do not have to search. You may be unable to stay with the master for a long time, but at least get yourself initiated, then you can practice on your own.

This will be your best use of money, time and effort.

Question

Once I was a bodybuilder and 3 times I hurt my back. I did many exercises and it helped but still I feel my back hurts like a "toothache". I believe that there is an exercise which restores the back, something like the Horse-Riding Stance, maybe static or active.

What should I do first, power exercises or flexibility?

Igal, USA (November 1999)

Answer

Your back still hurts because what you did were only physical exercises which only relieved your symptom temporary, and that symptom is pain. The cause of the problem, which is energy blockage, remains. To overcome the cause you have to do energy exercises, i.e. chi kung exercises.

Almost any chi kung exercise that "cleanses" can solve your problem. The Horse-Riding Stance and most power development methods are chi kung exercises that "build", and are therefore not suitable.

You may attain flexibility through physical exercises, but it may aggravate your problem, or at best only remove the symptom. Flexibility attained through chi kung will solve your problem.

Question

Can I learn and practice without direct supervision from a good master? Can videos and books help?

Chris, USA (October 2000)

Answer

You can learn from videos and books and practice without the supervision of a master, but it is certain that you will not get the best results; you may not even get mediocre results. Videos and books are helpful in showing you the outward forms of the practice, but not the inner essence.

If you think that just knowing the outward forms can lead to good kungfu and spiritual development, it is an indication you still have not understood what kungfu and spiritual development are.

Even at its basic, physical level, kungfu deals with combat, which necessitates skills like correct spacing, precise timing and versatility of movements.

Spiritual development deals with purifying the mind or spirit. Do you think videos and books can effectively deal with such matters?

Question

In your book, you mentioned that in the end it is force and not technique which would weigh more. I myself am not physically endowed, at 5'11", I weigh around 124 pounds. You could probably imagine how slim I am.

Force-wise, so far, I do not have much. I was under the impression that kungfu techniques would outweigh force, that force without direction was vulnerable to good techniques.

Jimmy, USA (May 1999)

Answer

There is a kungfu saying that is as follows;

- 1   li bu sheng quan
- 2   quan bu sheng gong
- 3   gong bu sheng guai
- 4   guai bu sheng jiao

Literally translated it is as follows:

- 1   strength is no match for technique
- 2   technique is no match for force
- 3   force is not match for speed
- 4   speed is no match for the marvelous

It means that in combat someone who has only brutal strength is no match for someone who applies kungfu techniques. For example, a physically stronger person may attack you with his "buffalo's strength", but if you use techniques effectively, such as stepping aside and then striking his ribs, you can defeat him. This is the first level of kungfu, and is the level you referred to in your question.

At the next level, you may use beautiful techniques and may actually strike your opponent many times, but unless the strikes are at vital spots like his eyes or genitals, if he is enormously forceful a single strike by him may be enough to fell you.

An interesting example is when a child holding the rank of black-belt spars with a forceful adult. Protected by safety rules and basing on points, the child would defeat the adult in a no-contact sparring competition, but in a real fight he will be no match for the adult.

Actually "force" here is a poor translation for the Chinese term "gong" (pronounced as "kung"). "Gong" includes not only force but also the ability to apply techniques skillfully.

The third level, the level after techniques and force, is speed. You must be fast enough to reach your opponent. It is worthy to note that while speed is the crucial factor at this level, you must have some basic techniques and force. If you are only fast, but have no techniques and no force, you may not be effective.

This serves as good advice to those practicing taijiquan and other "soft" arts like judo and aikido who mistakenly think that force is not needed in their arts, and what they need to defeat their opponents are good techniques and speed.

Force is needed in all martial arts; what is needed in these "soft" arts is "soft" force, and not "hard" force as in karate and taekwondo.

Take note that in the famous kungfu saying "four tahils or ounces of force to defeat one thousand katis or pounds of force", the exponent still needs at least four tahils of force. If he has only three tahils of force, it would be insufficient.

At the highest level, the decisive factor for victory is what is known as the marvelous, which is usually attained only by masters. It suggests that the master is so good that what he does is just right, and the opponent is simply overwhelmed.

For example just when the opponent thinks he has used a fantastic technique to defeat the master, he suddenly finds his technique being neutralized. When he thinks he is forceful, he finds that seemingly without much effort the master overcomes him. When he thinks he is fast, he finds he does not even know where the master's moves are coming from.

Question

I have been training for almost 6 months now and so far my Sifu's emphasis is technique and that force training will be later which I understand.

My concern is if force indeed is the determining factor then I will really have to do something like weight lifting, which I have tried before and really not my cup of tea.

Am I concerned about something trivial?
Jimmy, USA (May 1999)

Answer

Force training is essential in kungfu training, but it does not normally involve weight training in the western concept. In fact, such weight training is detrimental in traditional kungfu training. The later chapters will explain why this is so.

Perhaps what your sifu meant was specialized force training like Iron Palm or Iron Shirt. These arts of specialized force training should come after you are well versed in fundamental kungfu techniques.

Question

How should I balance the chi kung and kungfu training?
Raymond, Ireland (October 1998)

Answer

Chi kung is an integral part of genuine kungfu training. Chi kung means energy training. It is difficult to imagine any good kungfu without energy training.

Here I am referring to genuine chi kung, which involves a management of energy, and not to some debased chi kung form which is no more than gentle gymnastics or dance.

Question

Should I combine them in one session?
Raymond, Ireland (October 1998)

Answer

Yes. Kungfu without chi kung, or energy training, is low level kungfu. On the other hand, chi kung can be practiced on its own.

Question

How would the gentleness of chi kung followed by the 'explosiveness' of kungfu (one leaving me refreshed, while the other leaving me breathless!) affect the benefits of the chi kung exercises
Raymond, Ireland (October 1998)

Answer

There are different types of chi kung and also different types of kungfu. Some types of chi kung, like Iron Shirt and Sinew Metamorphosis, can be explosive, and some types of kungfu like Yang Style Taijiquan and Cotton Palm, can be gentle. But no chi kung or kungfu, irrespective of their types, irrespective of whether they are explosive or gentle, should leave you breathless if practiced correctly.

If you incorporate the right type of chi kung, such as one involving breath control, into an explosive type of kungfu such as Cannon Fist, you can execute the vigorous, explosive kungfu movements and forcefully without panting for breaths.

How would explosive kungfu affect the benefits of chi kung practice would depend on how you perform them. If you do them incorrectly, explosive kungfu might undo the chi kung benefits, such as distorting the smooth flow of energy derived from the chi kung practice earlier.

If you perform them correctly, their benefits complement and enhance each other, such as adding impetus and momentum to the internal force developed earlier from chi kung practice.

Question

I find specially demanding the Horse-Riding Stance — today, I can only endure it for 84 or 86 seconds at a time. I will continue practicing it until I reach the goal established by you, sifu.
Luis, Mexico (March 2000)

Answer

The Horse-Riding Stance is the most important exercise in Shaolin Kungfu. Besides giving you a solid base, it builds a pearl of energy at your abdominal energy field, and helps you to tame your mind.

If you practice the stance mechanically, as many students do on their own, it becomes a torture. When you realize and directly experience that you are developing your energy and mind, as when guided by a master, your training becomes a subtle joy.

Question

How long one should practice the stances? As I mean here, do somebody still train the stances as they have practice for let say 2-3 years.
Hendry, Indonesia (April 2000)

Answer

There are various stances. Let us take the Horse-Riding Stance for an example. It is reputed that in the past Shaolin monks had to practice the Horse-Riding Stance for two or three years before they were taught any kungfu patterns. Such a demand for high standard would not be practical today.

When I first learnt kungfu from Uncle Righteousness, I had to practice the Horse-Riding Stance for a few months. Although this was far from what the Shaolin monks did in the past, it was a very tough demand.

Many students in other schools did not have to spend time over the Horse-riding Stance; they went straight to kungfu movements the very first day. The difference was one of approach. My tradition emphasized force training; most other schools emphasized kungfu forms.

My standard, in turn, was much lower than that demanded by my master. My students had to practice the Horse-Riding Stance for at least a few weeks, then they were asked to continue the practice on their own. The minimum time I demand from my students on the stance is 5 minutes. In the past it was the time taken for a joss stick to be burnt out, which was about half an hour. But most students today cannot sit on the stance properly for a minute.

For how long should one continue practicing the stance, depends on various factors. Two influential factors are his knowledge (or wisdom) concerning the stance, and his scale of values.

If he realizes that stance-training, or zhan zhuang, is probably the most important single exercise from which most masters have developed their internal force, and if he values combat efficiency and vitality, he may continue practicing the Horse-Riding or other stances for years.

If he, like most people, think that the stance is just a dull routine without any relevance to actual fighting, and if he values beautiful forms to demonstrate or to teach others, he may never practice the stance again once he has learnt it.

In my opinion, if you practice the stance daily for three months, you would have attained a reasonable standard in today's martial art context. If you continue practicing for a year, you would have achieved remarkable internal force, relative to most modern martial artists.

Question

I am currently attending Shaolin Kungfu and have been learning for almost a year. I have read your web-page and book and have a few questions to ask you, if you do not mind.

I have only started to spar recently and, although my forms are all right, I find that I end up bouncing around the hall trying to avoid kicks and punches. I have tried to apply the simplest parts of my forms to sparring only to lose my timing and, once, walked into a kick to receive two broken ribs!

Does timing only come with practice? Although we are taught attack combinations, no one actually tells us what is wrong with our sparring.

I did Tang Soo Do when I was little and it seems that everyone in the class reverts to karate-style punching and kicking when they spar, forgetting the kungfu they have learnt.

Is there a systematic way to apply our techniques better to sparring?
Ryan, England

Answer

The situation you are in is a typical case of people learning kungfu today.

It is hard to believe but true that 90% of people learning kung fu today, including in China, do not know how to use their kungfu skills and techniques in combat. Most revert to karate, taekwondo or kickboxing techniques, and many fight like children.

If you have read my web-pages, you would find this concern is a major theme I have often stressed, but it is a delicate issue and I do not want to offend many kungfu instructors.

The main problem is that the methodology linking set practice and free sparring is generally lost. Going straight from set practice to free sparring, which 90% of kungfu practitioners do, will result in cases similar to yours. It is not feasible to explain the methodology in a short e-mail, and it is difficult to learn it without a master's personal tuition.

Nevertheless I shall try my best to answer your questions. You may also have some useful information on kungfu combat if you refer to my web-page.

I am extremely lucky to have been trained in the traditional Shaolin way, whereby we have to go through numerous stages from set practice to free sparring so that eventually we can spar in typical kungfu way.

I hope to share this methodology with deserving students, and may plan an intensive course in Malaysia, but those who wish to participate need to be instructors or have practiced kungfu for at least three years.

Timing is a crucial factor in combat. Many people think that to win in a fight all you need is techniques. In fact timing is more important than techniques. There is a kungfu saying as follows:*bai fa bu ru yi kuai*, which means it is better to be fast than to learn hundreds of techniques. If you are fast enough to strike an opponent, it does not matter which technique you use.

On the other hand, even if you know a lot of techniques, they will be quite useless if you are too slow to use them. But timing is more than just speed. Sometimes if you are too fast, it can be detrimental.

Timing does come with practice, but you must practice methodically. If you practice haphazardly, as many students do, you will still end up bouncing about trying to avoid kicks and punches, although with experience and improved speed you may succeed in the avoiding.

But soon you would be out of breath and eventually you would still lose the combat, but even if you win you would be reverting to karate-style punches and kicks, forgetting about all the kungfu you have learnt.

Actually you are lucky to realize this pathetic situation after only a year; many others, including "masters", keep on this pathetic situation for life, and if they do not have the opportunities to test their sparring effectiveness, or ineffectiveness, they may imagine they are practicing a wonderful kungfu.

Those who have some inkling of their combat ineffectiveness would, in an attempt to cover their inadequacy, turn aggressive whenever sparring is suggested, or mystify kungfu as such a deadly art that sparring practice even among classmates is forbidden.

Genuine kungfu exponents are calm and gentle as they do not have to prove to others and, more importantly, themselves that they can fight, because they know they can.

Sparring using kungfu patterns must be learnt methodically and systematically, otherwise students will revert to the more simple karate-style punches and kicks, or to the most natural way of fighting as exhibited by children.

Kungfu fighting is not natural fighting; it has to be learnt and acquired, and to be practiced and practiced methodically and systematically until it has become second-nature.

There are many steps between set training and free sparring. Thus, if an instructor or even a "master" asks you to practice sparring just after the set training stage, you can reasonably suspect that he does not know the essential intermediate steps.

Set training is to familiarize you with the form and practice of kungfu techniques; free sparring is to put these techniques, as well as appropriate tactics and strategies and other combative factors like force, timing, spacing, judgment and decision—making into action against an opponent or opponents.

Many useful tactics and strategies have been generalized into kungfu principles like "using minimum force against maximum strength" and "avoiding his strength and attacking his weakness".

Methodologies like specific techniques, combat sequences and sparring sets are employed to train combative factors to prepare for free sparring.

As there are more things to learn and practice in kungfu than in other martial arts, it is logical that it takes more time. A kickboxer can fight reasonably well after training for six months, a karate or taekwondo exponent in three years, but a kung fu practitioner would need more time.

This does not mean that you cannot fight until after practicing kungfu for more than ten years — as some "masters" buying time to cover their inadequacy may suggest.

In fact if you have practiced genuine kungfu — any style of kungfu including taijiquan — for a year or two, you should be able to provide some decent defense against any assailant irrespective of which martial arts the assailant may use; otherwise you should examine whether your art is genuine kungfu.

Question

We train a lot on a sack with sand, hitting the air with dumb-bells, a lot of power exercises and also A LOT of FULL CONTACT fights. My friends took many honorable places in different national and world competitions.

But when we fight it looks just like a street fight. I feel that I am not getting any close to becoming a real kungfu fighter. I am trying to practice as you say in the book but some how it does not look like it will lead me into a real kungfu fight.

I cannot imagine myself blocking fast real hits even after a few years by practicing the forms with myself or even in the later steps with friends.

I would be honored if I could get your advice.

Igal, Israel (April 1998)

Answer

Your problem is a very common problem with many kungfu students all over the world, including in China.

You may be surprised that modern wushu students and instructors, including those who have won championships, would also fight like street fighters or worse still like children. "Sanda" competitions, which are supposed to be free sparring wushu competitions, resemble boxing; you can hardly see any wushu patterns in these competitions.

In fact "sanda" competitors actually and actively employ boxing techniques in their training. In other words, in their attempt to fight well, they look as a model not towards a classical kungfu master but towards a modern western boxing expert, and what they typically discuss are not how to use a tiger-claw or butterfly-palm but how to throw a jab or a hook punch.

Yet, it is true that kungfu — any style of kungfu including taijiquan — is exceedingly effective for combat. In other words, not only a genuine kungfu student can fight using typical kungfu patterns, but also his chances of winning the fight is better if he uses kungfu patterns and not patterns taken from karate, taekwondo, kickboxing or any other martial arts.

Then why the overwhelming majority of kungfu students and instructors today all over the world cannot spar with kungfu patterns? I myself do not like to believe it is true, but it is true: today the art of kungfu for combat is virtually lost — with very, very rare exceptions, and for various reasons these exceptional masters are not willing or prepared to teach. In the last 50 years, the norm of teaching and learning kungfu has been to perform kungfu sets.

When the Chinese government promoted wushu, the Chinese official name for kungfu, the aim was, and still is, to promote it as a sport, and not as a martial art.

Hence, for those trained in kungfu sets or modern wushu, it is no surprise that they cannot use kungfu to spar. The beautiful kungfu or wushu sparring you see in movies and demonstrations are prearranged; unfortunately you do not see them in real sparring or fighting.

Even learning kungfu forms from a book is daunting enough; unless you are already trained, learning kungfu sparring from a book is practically impossible. This is because what is involved is not techniques but skills.

In other words it is learning not just how to block a punch or avoid a kick, but more importantly how to judge correctly, move swiftly and respond with sufficient force according to some preferred kungfu patterns.

One may clumsily learn techniques from a good book, but to develop combative skills one needs the personal supervision of a master.

I do not mean to sound presumptuous but I sincerely believe that I am one of the very few who have inherited the art of combat kungfu from the rare masters. Perhaps if the time is appropriate I may share this secret art with deserving students.

I must make it very clear that while I personally practice traditional kungfu, I do NOT disagree with the teaching and spread of wushu. Traditional kungfu and modern wushu have different aims and serve different needs.

Considering the situations today, I think the Chinese government has done a wonderful thing promoting wushu. The Chinese government has never pretended to spread combat kungfu; it has always explicitly emphasized the promotion of wushu as a sport because that best serves the needs of the present Chinese population.

Question

At our school we never do any serious sparring because my instructor believes doing set practice will give us a better understanding of the techniques.
Jason, USA (November 1999)

Answer

I strongly disagree with your instructor's view. Set practice enables you to perform kungfu techniques correctly and develop certain combat skills, but without sparring practice you can never be competent in self-defense.

Even practicing sparring sets (where whole sets consist of prearranged sparring patterns between two or more persons) is insufficient.

In other words, if you only do set practice you may understand the techniques in theory, but if you are caught in a combat situation you will be unable to use the techniques in actual fighting.

Question

What are your thoughts on sparring and the use of boxing gloves while sparring ?
Jason, USA (November 1999)

Answer

To be able to swim, you must practice swimming; to be able to play football, you must practice playing football. To be able to spar, you must practice sparring.

If you just learn swimming techniques on land, or learn football techniques in a classroom, but without practicing the techniques in a pool or a field, you will never be able to swim or play football.

Similarly if you just learn kungfu techniques in set practice, but without practicing the techniques in sparring, you will never be able to use the techniques to fight, although you may understand their uses theoretically and be able to demonstrate them beautifully in solo performance to please spectators.

Past masters called such kungfu demonstrative forms "flowery fists and embroidery kicks".

From my experiences, I can reasonably say that instructors or even "masters" who teach sparring with the use of boxing gloves, cannot competently apply their kungfu techniques for combat.

They and their students usually spar or fight like western boxers or kickboxers. I wonder if you have seen any kungfu or wushu sparring competitions, now called "san-da" in Chinese. They are a disgrace to the art.

These competitors punch and kick like boxers, and bounce about the ring like boxers, having thrown kungfu features like the tiger-claw or the bow-arrow stance to the winds.

Question

How much time do you recommend that I should spend on forms and set practice compared to sparring ?
Jason, USA (November 1999)

Answer

You should spend at least 50% of the time on not just sparring, but sparring using kungfu techniques. This cannot be learnt from books or videos; it has to be taught and guided by a competent instructor.

You may have learnt various kungfu techniques well in set practice and think that you know their combat applications, but it is only in sparring that they come to life, and you will be amazed at the beauty and efficiency of kungfu techniques in comparison to straight-forward punching, kicking and blocking.

Question

How much time do your students spend on sparring compared to set practice and do they use boxing gloves and other such protective gears?
Jason, USA (November 1999)

Answer

About 30% on set practice and 70% on sparring. Many of the sets they practice are composed by themselves from the combat sequences taught by me or sometimes developed by themselves from their sparring practice. Hence, apart from basic sets which provide the repertoire of their sparring sequences, different students practice different sets of their own.

We do not use boxing gloves or other protective gears like groin guards, knee pads or cushion mats. When my students first learn felling techniques, when they let their partners throw them to the ground, they practice in a field if it is available. Later, when they know how to counter throws they practice on hard ground.

Question

I am feeling very disillusioned about my kungfu practice, what's the use of training so hard if I cannot use what I have learnt to defend myself...
Jason, USA (November 1999)

Answer

You are in a minority regarding disillusion, but in a great majority regarding the inability to defend yourself. Probably more than 90% of people all over the world, including in China, who say they do kungfu or wushu, and this includes Taijiquan, cannot use what they learnt in set practice to defend themselves.

If we leave out Taijiquan, the proportion is still very high, probably more than 75%. Many of them can defend themselves, but not using kungfu or wushu; they frequently use boxing, taekwondo or kickboxing.

Most of them have not reached the stage of disillusion — they are still at the stage of illusion. Some of them honestly think they are doing wonderful kungfu, and some actively promote it, sitting in influential committees of kungfu organizations.

Question

You said that you do not believe in the use of boxing gloves for sparring. How then do your students manage to spar without hurting each other.
Jason, USA (December 1999)

Answer

It is illuminating to note that not a single kungfu master in the past used boxing gloves when sparring with other masters, sparring with his students, or when teaching his students sparring, and they did not hurt each other. Boxing gloves are meant for boxing or kickboxing, not for kungfu.

Karate, taekwondo, jujitsu, judo, aikido and hapkido do not use boxing gloves, and when their exponents spar, onlookers could tell their style from their sparring.

It is only in modernized, and often greatly modified, kungfu that boxing gloves are used, and when these kungfu exponents spar, they spar like boxers or kickboxers, or worse still like children.

My personal opinion is that, apart from special occasions, anyone — including a master — who uses boxing gloves in teaching sparring does not know how to use genuine kungfu techniques in combat, even though he may be a good fighter (using non-kungfu techniques).

Not only my students do not use boxing gloves for sparring, they do not have any special protection like knee-guards and groin-guards, and they spar on hard floors. Yet, serious injury resulting from sparring is nil. This is due to the following reasons.

1. They are fully aware that the purpose of sparring is to mutually help each other to improve combat skills, and not to out-do each other. Hence if one finds his partner too slow, he will purposely slow down his attack to accommodate his partner.

   If he strikes his partner, this will end that part of their sparring practice, giving them no chance to proceed further. If he purposely slows down, he experiences one of those rare occasions when he can more perceptively observe how an opponent moves, thereby noticing weaknesses which he can exploit if he wants to.

2. They have good control of their attack. They employ what is known in kungfu terminology as "dian dow wei zi" (or "tim tou wai tze" in Cantonese), which is "contact by merely touching gently".

3. Their approach to sparring is systematic and methodical. They never jump into free sparring immediately. They go through numerous stages of prearranged sparring, then semi-free sparring so that by the time they practice free sparring they can effectively defend themselves.

   Unlike in most other martial art schools where free sparring is the beginning and end of sparring, and where practitioners go in freely to punch and kick each other, in traditional Shaolin training, free sparring is the accumulation of a long series of various sparring practices, where practitioners test out and confirm — rather than practice — their combat efficiency.

   In other words, in traditional Shaolin training, students (and masters too) do not use free sparring to practice combat; rather, they use free sparring to confirm that they are combat efficient.

But injuries sometimes occur, even in prearranged sparring, but they are usually not serious. They can be overcome in literally five minutes by performing appropriate chi kung exercises, especially "Lifting the Sky". This solves about 80% of the injuries.

In the other 20%, I open the relevant energy points of an injured student, transmit some chi into him and ask him to perform a spontaneous chi flow exercise. In about 15 minutes his injury would be overcome.

On very rare occasions, I have to prescribe some kungfu medicine for an injured student to apply externally and take in orally. He would recover in one to three weeks.

In my kungfu training days I was once injured seriously. I was free sparring with my siheng, or senior classmate, who was even smaller-sized than I was. He gave me a double-punch; I gripped his two wrists with double tiger-claws, immobilizing his attack.

In my inexperience I thought that was the completion of a practice sequence. But he meant his attack to be a trap. He released my grips with a twist of his wrists and struck my solar plexus with a cup-fist at close quarters.

Seeing that I could not defend the unexpected attack, he pulled back immediately, merely touching my chest with the fist.

Even for just a tap, he was sincerely sorry. I still remember that he said he thought I knew how to counter the attack because it was found in our Shaolin Pakua Set. I told him I had learnt the set but had not learnt that particular application. We thought nothing about the gentle tap; there was not even any mark on my skin, nor any pain.

But a few days later my eyes turned yellowish, and I could hardly speak. I knew immediately that I had sustained internal injury from my siheng's tap. I told my sifu, and he confirmed the injury. My siheng's internal force was so powerful that it distorted the energy field in my chest and caused some serious energy blockage.

My sifu applied some external medicine on my chest, and prescribed some internal medicine for me to drink. After a few days, my chest turned purplish black, as a result of the medication drawing out "dead blood" from my internal injury.

It took me three months of medication and remedial chi kung exercise to recover. Should anyone think that internal force is a myth, I can vouch from my personal and direct experience that it is true. Understandably many people will find it outlandish; I myself might not believe it if not for my own experience.

My siheng did not even strike me; he actually pulled back his punch. I reckon that if my siheng struck an opponent's solar plexis, especially with a phoenix-eye fist instead of a cup-fist, that person would die — not immediately, but after a few months, and he might not even know why.

This experience was an invaluable lesson to me — learnt first hand. Subsequently in my numerous sparring sessions and occasional fights, I made doubly sure I was safe before I released my guard.

Gradually I became so intuitively perceptive that later, on many occasions when I paused to explain finer points to my students during sparring but they unintentionally continued to strike me, I could still ward off their attacks.

Question

The sparring we do is not sparring in the true sense of the word. We are attacked once with any type of attack and we are expected to use the techniques we have learnt to defend ourselves.
Jason, USA (December 1999)

Answer

This is one-step sparring, and is usually used at the beginning of learning to spar. But your approach is haphazard. In this case the defender will often be uncertain and hesitant.

A better approach is as follows. Decide on only one type of attack, and the defender knows what technique to use to defend against this pre-chosen attack. Practice this one-step pre-chosen attack and defense at least ten times before changing to another type of attack and defense.

The onus of this training is not learning to use which technique to defend against an attack, but to develop the necessary skills like judgment, spacing and timing in using a pre-chosen defense appropriate for that particular type of attack.

Anyone with some experience of fighting will know that skills are much more important than techniques. This is probably the most important factor why kungfu practitioners today are generally no match against karate or taekwondo exponents. They know, in theory, hundreds of techniques but they have no skills to use even the simplest of techniques effectively.

Question

Currently I am practicing about 3-4 times a week, I want to get more serious about my practice. What is the maximum amount of time one should spend per week to get optimal results?
Jason, USA (December 1999)

Answer

Maximum time and optimal results are philosophical concepts. In practice, they vary greatly from individuals to individuals and from situations to situations. Variables like knowledge and exposure, needs and abilities, resources and instructions are influential.

The maximum time and optimal results of someone who uses boxing gloves and hopes to match up to a karate black-belt are very different from those of another who emulates the classical kungfu masters.

If you use boxing gloves and training methods generally employed by most kungfu schools today, and if you train for two hours per session about 3-4 times a week, you can fight in six months, and can take on a black-belt in three years.

But if continue training for 30 years you will not be much better in fighting; you may even be worse due to your advancing age.

If you follow traditional kungfu methods which are rare nowadays and which do not use boxing gloves, and if you train for two hours per session about 3-4 times a week, you cannot fight in six months, but you can handle a black-belt comfortably in three years.

If you continue training for 30 years you can handle a black-belt like a child, and you will have better health and vitality than when you began training 33 years ago.

As most people today are so used to kungfu that has been much modernized and modified that it serves the purpose of gymnastics and dance more than a combat art, they will find it hard to believe how a traditional kungfu master can handle a black-belt like a child.

Indeed the opposite situation is more common. Many masters teaching modernized kungfu, such as wushu and tai chi where sparring is never a part of their training, may be quite helpless when attacked by black-belts.

But you may have a good idea if you look at it this way. After 30 years of training where internal force and sparring are crucial components, the traditional kungfu master will have become extremely powerful and have gone through millions of times combative movements black-belts typically use.

The attacks of a black-belt, while damaging to the uninitiated, are actually quite straight-forward. Hence when a black-belt attacks him, the traditional kungfu master merely handles the attacks as if they are part of his daily training routine.

Wushu

Question

How does modern Chinese wushu (such as that taught at the Shaolin Monastery) differ from "traditional" kungfu?

Karl, Sweden (July 1998)

Answer

The term "wushu" actually means "martial art", i.e. what in the West would be referred to as kungfu.

However, the present Chinese government has explicitly stated that it is promoting wushu as a sport and not as a martial art.

This then is the crucial difference. Modern wushu is a sport, whereas traditional kungfu is a martial art. Logically if you practice modern wushu as a sport, you will get benefits which sports generally give, such as keeping fit and healthy, recreation, opportunities to compete within certain rules, and public demonstration.

Since modern wushu is originally derived from traditional kungfu, you may, after considerable guidance from a kungfu master and further practice on your own, apply the dance-like wushu movements for self-defense. But by itself, modern wushu is not capable for combat, simply because its training is not meant for such a purpose.

If you match a world wushu champion, for example, against a karate black-belt or a western style boxer, it is most likely that the wushu champion will be beaten badly. If you compare the demonstration of wushu against that of karate or western boxing, there is, in my opinion, nothing in karate, western boxing or any other martial arts or sports that can match the superb elegance and beauty of wushu movements.

Traditional kungfu is fundamentally a martial art, i.e. its training is geared towards combat. However, for various reasons, many schools that teach traditional kungfu today may not be able to use traditional kungfu movements for self-defense. If such exponents have to fight, they usually use techniques borrowed from other martial systems, particularly from karate, taekwondo and kickboxing.

If you match exponents of karate, western boxing or other martial systems against genuine kungfu exponents, basing on purely theoretical principles, the kungfu exponents will win, although in real life this may not be true because there are many other practical factors involved besides theoretical considerations.

If history can be of any indication, kungfu is superior to other martial arts; virtually all masters of various martial arts from many countries, such as Japan, Korea, Russia and France, who went to China to test her kungfu masters in the early twentieth century, were convincingly defeated.

Great kungfu like Shaolin and Taijiquan is more than merely a martial art. It is a complete and comprehensive program for physical, emotional, mental and spiritual cultivation, leading to the highest attainment any person can ever attain, called variously as enlightenment, unity with the Cosmos or return to God.

Question

There are wushu instructors who insist that their art is also directly from the Shaolin Temple. Without a genuine point of reference such as that which you can provide, many enthusiasts will also be mistaken.

I know that these instructors are wushu exponents because they confirm their adequacy by mentioning their membership in wushu teams in mainland China, bronze medal awards, etc.

Marlene, Australia (January 2000)

Answer

Modern wushu is not Shaolin Kungfu. In the 1960s the Chinese government gathered together some kungfu masters from various styles with the objective of synthesizing the various styles into one uniform style, which is today's modern wushu.

Prior to that, there were numerous kungfu styles like Lohan, Praying Mantis, Eagle Claw, Chaquan, Huaquan, Hoong Ka, Wing Chun, Hsing Yi, Pa Kua, etc. After that, there was to be no differentiation into these various styles, only wushu.

Wushu was invented solely for sports, and never as a martial art. For the purpose of competition, wushu was divided into seven categories, namely,

- 1   Changquan, or Long Fist
- 2   Nanquan or Southern Fist
- 3   Daoshu or Knife Techniques
- 4   Jianshu or Sword Techniques
- 5   Kunshu or Staff Techniques
- 6   Chiangshu or Spear Techniques
- 7   Taijiquan or Tai Chi Chuan

The sole criterion for the award of points in all wushu competitions is how graceful and elegant the performance is, and never how well a performer can defend himself or how much internal force he has.

The wushu instructors were quite right to say that wushu was derived from Shaolin Kungfu because except for Taijiquan and aerobatic movements, virtually all wushu movements were taken from Shaolin Kungfu. But their statement is misleading, as their nature and purposes are very different.

Question

Also, a kungfu master insisted that Chinese martial arts are all called wushu; kungfu is only a Cantonese term meaning hard work.
Marlene, Australia (January 2000)

Answer

From one perspective he is right, but from another perspective — the one we are using now — he is wrong. The sameness or difference between kungfu and wushu has confused many people, but the following explanation will clear the confusion.

Kungfu, used in the sense of Chinese martial art, has many terms in the Chinese language. The present official term is "wushu". Besides this term, another term that is most commonly used for what in the West would be conceptualized as "kungfu" is "quanfa", often shortened to "quan". Thus, Shaolin Kungfu is "shaolinquan" or "shaolin wushu" in Chinese, and Tai Chi Kungfu is "taijiquan" or "taiji wushu".

It is also true that in Cantonese, as well as many other Chinese dialects including Mandarin, "kungfu" literally means "work". But today when a person uses the word "kungfu", he usually means "martial art", using the term "kung-chok" for "work".

Complications started when the present Chinese government promoted newly invented modern wushu as a sport, and not as a marital art. The trend has been so established that today when the term "wushu" is used, especially in the West, it is conceptualized as a demonstrative sport, whereas when the term "kungfu" is used it is conceptualized as a martial art.

In other words, we now have an interesting situation whereby although the word "wushu" literally means "martial art", in practical usage it is a demonstrative sport; and although the word "kungfu" literally means "work", it is a martial art.

To say that all Chinese martial arts are wushu is like saying all persons are men, insisting that the word "mankind" refers to humankind.

Question

I have seen actors like Jet Li. What kind of kungfu did he master? Is it wushu?

Alvin, Singapore (October 1999)

Answer

Jet Li is a wushu master. His wushu is magnificent, and he has won national championships in China many times.

What Jet Li and other actors like him show in movies is beautiful Shaolin Kungfu. But, unfortunately, such beautiful kungfu application very seldom happens in real life sparring.

Today when kungfu students spar, usually they are unable to apply the beautiful kungfu techniques they have learnt, and therefore have to resort to simple kicks and punches.

Traditional Weapons

Question

Could you please give more information about the many weapons of Shaolin Kungfu?

Darren, UK (April 2000)

Answer

Shaolin Kungfu, especially Northern Shaolin, is exceeding rich in weapons.

In the past weapon training was more important than unarmed training.

This was logical because, except for the unrealistic heroes that we normally see in the movies, who would not use a weapon in combat when weapons could be carried about freely.

Since the Yuan or Mongolian Dynasty, however, when weapons were outlawed, unarmed fighting became more prominent.

Shaolin weapons were traditionally divided into two main categories: long and short.

Long weapons are those with the weapon head attached to a long staff, such as the spear, the battle axe, the Big Knife, the Big Trident, and the snake-lance.

Short weapons are held by a short handle in one hand, such as the knife, the sword, the rod, the soft whip, and the dagger.

The kungfu saying, "one inch longer, one inch stronger; one inch shorter, one inch trickier", summarizes the comparative advantage of the long and the short weapons.

If you hold a long spear, for example, you can more easily keep your opponent at bay. If you hold a dagger, especially when you have succeeded in getting close to your opponent, you have a greater range of techniques.

The most important, as well as most representative of both Northern and Southern Shaolin weapons, is the staff.

It looks simple but all the important techniques of long weapons as well as most of the techniques of short weapons are found in it! The staff is therefore considered as both a long as well as short weapon.

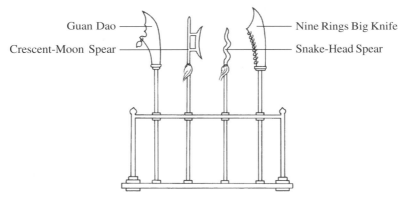

Guan Dao ——⟶ — Nine Rings Big Knife

Crescent-Moon Spear ——⟶ — Snake-Head Spear

Traditional Chinese Weapons

Question
Which weapons are common to certain styles and which weapons you practice/teach?
Darren, UK (April 2000)

Answer
The most popular weapons common to most styles are the knife (or broadsword), the sword, the staff and the spear. Hence, these four are the only weapons found in modern wushu.

Some styles are well known for particular weapons.

Some examples are the single knife of Hoong Ka, the butterfly knives of Wing Chun, the big-knife of Choy-Li-Fatt, the three-section staff of Praying Mantis, and the tiger-hooks of Eagle Claw Kungfu. In the internal styles, Taijiquan is famous for the sword, Baguazhang for the single knife, and Xingyi for the spear.

I used to practice and teach a great variety of weapons, including more fanciful ones like the soft whip, the copper hammer, the snake-lance and the crescent-moon spade.

But in my more matured years, I have discarded much of teaching weapons and focused on unarmed combat, realizing that although practicing with kungfu weapons still bring present-day benefits, in realistic terms it is more for demonstrations.

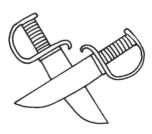

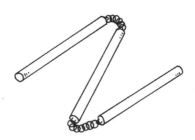

Butterfly Knives   Three-Sectional Staff

Question

Also could you demonstrate an application of the three section staff and double tiger hooks?
Darren, UK (April 2000)

Answer

I am not trained in the three-section staff or the double tiger-hooks, and thus would not be able to give a good demonstration. I would instead demonstrate a wrong, but common, application of two weapons I know quite well — the staff and the sword — and how they should be used.

Question

I would like to know your expert knowledge on the Southern Shaolin broadsword.
Damila, USA (April 2000)

Answer

As there is there is not much difference between the Southern Shaolin broadsword and the broadsword of other kungfu styles, I shall discuss the broadsword in general.

The term "broadsword" has become an established term for the kungfu weapon which the Chinese call "dao", or "tou" in Cantonese pronunciation. Personally I prefer to call it "knife", which is a more literal translation of the Chinese word "dao", although in English it may connote a cutting implement rather than a weapon.

I choose "knife" instead of "broadsword" because I wish to focus on a crucial distinction between a knife or "dao" and a sword or "jian" in kungfu philosophy and practice. A knife has only one cutting edge whereas both edges of a sword can be used for cutting.

More important is the way these two different weapons are used. Using a sword as if it were a knife, as it was frequently the case in many of the crowd-drawing Hong Kong movies in the 1960s featuring classical swordsmen, is a clear indication that the swordsman does not know the art of genuine swordsmanship.

A sword is to be used as a sword, and a knife as a knife. Their techniques and skills are quite different. Using a sword like a knife is sure to have the sword broken into many pieces. On the other hand, using a knife like a sword would result in losing the ferocious qualities of the knife, for which it is intended.

Interestingly, the samurai sword, from the kungfu perspective, is a knife and not a sword. Using a knife instead of a sword would be in line with the nature and work of a samurai.

What many people may not know is that the samurai sword was introduced to Japan from China during the Ming Dynasty, when many Ming warriors used a heavy sharp weapon known as "willow-leaf knife", held with both hands like what kendo practitioners nowadays do.

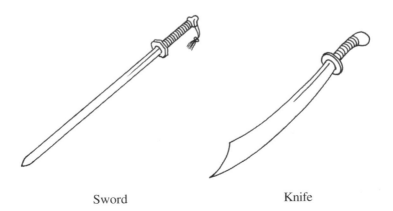

Sword   Knife

Question

What are the internal and external characteristics of the Southern Shaolin broadsword?

Damila, USA (April 2000)

Answer

Whether the characteristics are internal or external depends on relative and often arbitrary interpretations. But a good principle to use when making a differentiation is the kungfu tenet: "internally train jing, shen and qi, and externally train jin, gu and pi", which means internal arts focus on the training of essence, mind and energy, whereas external arts focus on the training of muscles, bones and flesh.

Hence, if you perform stance-training, meditation, and breath control, yours are internal characteristics; if you stretch your muscles, strengthen your bones, and toughen your flesh, such as skipping and hitting sandbags, yours are external characteristics.

The kungfu knife or broadsword as well as all other weapons involve both internal and external training. I am referring to knife training in genuine kungfu. If one merely performs the outward forms of a knife set, then it is external. But if in performing the set, he does so in a heightened state of consciousness and regulates his breathing accordingly, it is also internal.

Some important internal characteristics of the kungfu knife exponent are being ferocious like a tiger, focusing the mind exactly as he makes a defense or an attack move, channeling his energy flow to the sharp blade of the weapon, and regulating his breathing appropriately.

If he, for example, performs his kungfu knife movements as if he is doing an Indian club demonstration, or close his mouth tight when making a powerful chop, he would have missed the internal characteristics — irrespective of whether his kungfu knife is from Southern Shaolin or other styles.

The external characteristics include all the techniques of the kungfu knife, which are explained below, as well as combative factors like footwork, speed, balance and fluidity of movements.

Question

What are some of the Southern Shaolin broadsword sets?
Damila, USA (April 2000)

Answer

As most kungfu styles have only one knife set, it is usually named after the style, such as Shaolin Single Knife, Shaolin Double Knives, Taiji Single Knife, Bagua Single Knife, Chow Ka Single Knife, and Wuzu Single Knife.

There is only one set because as the main purpose of the past masters was to use the knife for combat, and not to perform flowery sets to please spectators, just one knife set was sufficient for them to train the relevant knife skills and techniques for effective fighting.

There are, however, countless versions of any set. In other words, there is not just one set of Shaolin Single Knife; there may be hundreds of them — all having the same name but with different sequences and different patterns. This is because through the centuries the prototype set has been modified countless times by different masters to suit countless different situations and environments.

Nevertheless, two knife sets are well known in both Northern Shaolin and Southern Shaolin. They are "Plum Flow Single Knife" and "Sun and Moon Double Knives". But there are countless versions of these two famous knife sets.

Question

If you may, could you list the Cantonese and Mandarin names of the broadsword cuts and techniques?
Damila, USA (April 2000)

Answer

Here are the Chinese names (in Cantonese) and their English translations of common knife techniques:

1. Phat, Vertical Chop — chopping the knife downward in a vertical manner.
2. Cham, Slanting Chop — chopping the knife downward in a slanting manner.
3. Liew, Reversed Swing — swinging the knife upward with the sharp edge facing upward.
4. Sou, Horizontal Sweep — sweeping the sharp edge of the knife in a horizontal manner.

5. Kar, Upward Block — using the blunt edge or the side of the knife to block upward
6. Lan, Sideward Block — using the blunt edge or the side of the knife to block sideways.
7. Chee, Thrust — thrusting the pointed end of the knife forward.
8. Lai, Pull — slicing with the sharp edge of the knife.
9. Thiew, Flick — flicking the knife to one side with the blunt edge or with the sharp point.
10. Khoi, Cover — pushing down an opponent's weapon with the side of the knife.

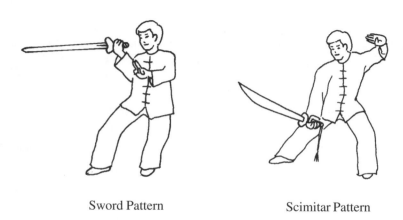

Sword Pattern   Scimitar Pattern

Question

What should we look for when buying a broadsword?
Damila, USA (April 2000)

Answer

If you intend to use it for demonstration, which is usually the case nowadays, the kungfu knife or broadsword should be light, shining and flabby so that it can make a clanging sound when you wield it.

If you intend to use it for fighting, which is actually not recommended, it should be fairly heavy and thick at its back (or the blunt side), tapering to this pointed end, and with a heavy nob at the end of the handle to balance the length of the knife. It should never be flabby, but it would make a "shsss" sound when it cuts through the air.

Taijiquan

The Practice Of Taiji Is A Daily Joy

Professor Javier Galve
a professor of computer science and a teacher of Taiji

I attended three Chi-kung courses with Sifu Wong before contacting him for a Taiji course. His Taiji web-page was the spark that lit up my mind.

Taiji as a martial art or as a way of developing internal force had been merely theory and nothing else for me. I felt for a long time that my Taiji had been lacking something like that.

I took advantage of one of his visits to Spain and phoned him. Sifu scheduled a ten-day course in Malaysia and we went ahead with it in summer(1998).

Once in Malaysia, I had one of the most profound experiences in my life. Besides the impact of such a beautiful country, the teachings of Sifu Wong and the knowledge that he gave me turned around my previous eight years of Taiji practice.

The sessions consisted of hard work. The first days, we spent some time correcting the stances and the Taiji patterns that I had learnt incorrectly. Sifu pointed out that my back was bent and it was true that I frequently had back pains (I had the beginnings of scoliosis).

Every day, after the Taiji form, Sifu let the Self-Manifested Chi Movement work in my body. I felt a "healthy pain" in my back and in my legs. I particularly remember one session when I spent about one hour in a very special state of mind. I passed through various stages.

My body moved in circles at first and then forward and backward. After that, I began to feel like a snake, and I even saw internally (don't ask me how) the point in my spine that was damaged.

Through the gift that Sifu has, he passed to me "from heart to heart," as he says, the knowledge and ability to clean chi blockages using Taiji to tap cosmic energy and how to see Taiji as a meditation technique. Because of that, I see Taiji as a way; a path to develop a "chi sensibility," which is like saying a "life sensibility."

After yin always comes yang. That is a wisdom message for daily life. Taiji makes every day, every time of practice and every movement a different experience. "Open your heart" was the phrase he told me at the beginning of the training session every day.

Feeling his advice, the practice of Taiji is a daily joy and that is something for which I shall always be grateful to Sifu Wong.

Madrid January 9th, 1999
Javier
Email jgalve@fi.upm.es

Teaching Me To Smile From The Heart

Jeffrey Segal, Musician, Switzerland

I do not think that I can find the right words to thank you properly but if I had to thank you for one thing it would definitely be for teaching me to smile from the heart. Just imagining you saying those words makes my spine straight, my mind empty and my heart radiant.

Dear Sifu,

So many things happen every day that make me think of you that I just feel like writing you an email to say thank you. My whole life seems more flowing and full of fun and things that used to upset me remind me of you saying the word "petty".

I think that my training is going well. I certainly enjoy it immensely. I hope from deep in my heart that we'll find some time for you to give courses in Zürich. Also, if you think that I am ready to be an instructor it will be my honor to give classes in your name.

I am reading your delightful "Complete Book of Tai Chi Chuan" again. What an inspiration! Thank you also for your fantastic web-site.

I do not know whether Taylor sent you the photo he took of us but I am attaching it to this e-mail. Just looking at this photo fills me with joy. I have sent it to my family and some friends and they all love it.

Laura also sent me some photos taken during our afternoon in Segovia. She calls me "lucky man" and I do feel extremely lucky to be your student.

I have been in contact with Adalia and I will be in Barcelona from the 27th till the 30th of October. I have also been e-mailing Linda and I have booked my flights for Malaysia in December. I am coming for the intensive Chi Kung course and the intensive Tai Chi Chuan course.

I do not think that I can find the right words to thank you properly but if I had to thank you for one thing it would definitely be for teaching me to smile from the heart. Just imagining you saying those words makes my spine straight, my mind empty and my heart radiant.

See you in Barcelona!

In deep respect and gratitude

Jeffrey Segal
E-mail: je.segal@active.ch.
21st September 2000

History

Question

I have been talking with my wife and we plan to take Tai Chi classes. I want to learn more about the history as well as the spiritual and mental aspects of the art.

What recommendations would you offer to a future student?

Robert, USA (September 1999)

Answer

First, decide whether you wish to practice Tai Chi dance or genuine Tai Chi Chuan. Tai Chi dance gives you benefits like balance and gracefulness, as well as recreation and socialization. Genuine Tai Chi Chuan gives you good health, vitality, combat efficiency, mental freshness and spiritual joy.

If you are contented with Tai Chi dance, it is easy to find an instructor, and its practice is generally easy and fun. Finding a genuine Tai Chi Chuan master is very difficult, practicing it is even more difficult, but the rewards are worth all the difficulties.

The history of Tai Chi dance is about fifty to a hundred years. There was no specific point in time when Tai Chi dance started, and there were no founders. Tai Chi dance developed, or more correctly degenerated from genuine Tai Chi Chuan perhaps about a hundred years ago, but it has gathered momentum very quickly in the last fifty years.

Today, as a rough estimate, more than 90% of those who practice Tai Chi, practices the degenerated dance version, and not the original genuine version. A notable factor is that those who practice Tai Chi dance usually do not know they are doing so; they think they are doing genuine Tai Chi Chuan.

A simple, effective way to find out whether yours is Tai Chi dance or Tai Chi Chuan is as follows. As genuine Tai Chi Chuan is an internal martial art, you can find out by checking whether your have learnt (or will learn) anything internal and martial in your art. If you are not sure, then you have not learnt them; if you had, you will surely know.

Tai Chi Chuan has a history of more than seven hundred years. Its "founder" was the great Taoist priest Zhang San Feng, who evolved it from Shaolin Kungfu. It was first called Wudang Long Fist. Later the scholar-general Chen Wang Ting called it Tai Chi Chuan, which means "Cosmos Kungfu".

There is nothing much that can be considered spiritual or mental in Tai Chi dance. Although in theory many Tai Chi dance instructors may say that their art is rich in Taoist philosophies which pays much attention to the spirit or mind, in practice virtually all their attention is given to physical matters, like how to coordinate your hands and legs, and how to move gracefully.

On the other hand, genuine Tai Chi Chuan training involves cultivating the "three treasures", namely jing, qi and shen, which are matter, energy and spirit or mind. Indeed, every movement in genuine Tai Chi Chuan is a training of energy and mind.

Taijiquan for Health and Self-Defense

Question

I am somehow confused with the fact that you said Taijiquan was a martial art, but here in Singapore I do not see anyone practicing it as a form of kungfu but with some swords.

Is wushu, Taijiquan, Shaolin Kungfu and Xingyiquan the same?

Alvin, Singapore (October 1999)

Answer

Taijiquan is (or at least was) definitely a martial art. "Quan" in "Taijiquan" is the shortened form for "quan-fa", which is one of many Chinese terms for martial art, or what in English is usually referred to as kungfu.

Other examples include "Shaolinquan" (Shaolin Kungfu), Xingyiquan (Hsing Yi Kungfu), Chaquan (Cha Kungfu) and Luohanquan (Lohan Kungfu).

Wushu is another Chinese term for martial art. It is now officially used by the present Chinese government. In Taiwan, the official term for Chinese martial art is guoshu.

Taijiquan, Shaolin Kungfu and Xingyiquan are different forms of wushu, or in more familiar English terms, different forms of kungfu. But because the present Chinese government has standardized various ancient forms of wushu into one modern version, and promotes it as sport, the term "wushu" is often used today to denote a modern form of kungfu movements quite distinct from traditional kungfu forms such as Taijiquan, Shaolin Kungfu and Xingyiquan.

The lamentable thing is that not only Taijiquan but all other forms of kungfu are rarely practiced as martial art. They have been debased into gymnastics or dance.

Although these arts may still be called Taijiquan, Shaolin Kungfu, etc., by their practitioners, they are not the genuine Taijiquan, Shaolin Kungfu, etc., they used to be in the past.

Practitioners of some styles of kungfu may still spar, but what they use in their sparring is usually not what they have learnt in their solo practice but borrowed from other martial systems like karate, taekwondo and kickboxing.

Question

Can you explain the structure of Taijiquan?

I have basic knowledge of the difference between the Chen and Yang style, short and long but I also saw videos on the 24 forms, the 32 forms, etc.

Ron, USA (December 1998)

Answer

There are a few ways to approach this topic. One way is to approach Taijiquan, or any kungfu, from the perspectives of form, energy and mind. Basically, you use the form to develop energy and mind.

The form can be mobile, such as the 24-pattern set or the 36-pattern set you mention; or static, such as zhan zhuang using the Three-Circle Stance or jing-zao which is silent sitting.

When you move an arm in a moving form, for example, you focus your mind and direct your energy to flow along the arm to the fingers. When you remain in zhan zhuang, you expand your mind and increase your energy level.

Another way is to approach from the perspectives of form, force, application and philosophy. Basically, with an understanding of the philosophy of Taijiquan, you employ form to develop force for combat as well as everyday application.

For example, from its philosophy if you appreciate that Taijiquan is an internal martial art, which many people pay lip service to but do not really understand, you will realize that you cannot be practicing genuine Taijiquan if what you do, does not contribute to internal cultivation and combat efficiency.

Roughly speaking Chen Style Taijiquan is more conducive to combat efficiency, and Yang Style Taijiquan to health promotion. This, of course, does not means that Chen Style does not contribute to health, nor Yang Style is not effective for combat.

The 24-pattern set and the 36-pattern set are just two of the many tools one can use to achieve the aims and objectives of Taijiquan. One can be proficient in Taijiquan without having to know these two sets. In fact not a single great Taijiquan master in the past knew any one of these sets because these sets were invented only recently.

But these sets are very useful — if you know how to use them correctly. They can help you to become proficient in Taijiquan in a shorter time had you followed the older, orthodox sets.

The big problem is that many people who say they practice Taijiquan do not know how to use these sets correctly. Instead of using them as tools to develop energy and mind, or to develop internal force for combat and everyday application, they regard them as ends by themselves.

They mistakenly think that Taiji form, which constitutes only a part of Taijiquan, as the whole of Taijiquan. As a result they become Taiji dancers, or at best Taiji gymnasts, instead of genuine Taijiquan exponents.

To be fair, the fault often is not entirely theirs. People in general do not appreciate, or refuse to accept, the fact that genuine Taijiquan or any kungfu style was, is and will be rare; and even if one has the rare opportunity to learn from a real master, he has to put in a lot, a lot and a lot of hard work.

The situation today, especially in the west, is that one thinks he can, without any prior experience, learn genuine Taijiquan from a book or a video, and after three months start to teach it.

If a genuine master is kind enough to point out his mistakes, he regards it an insult; if he is asked to bow to his master, he thinks it outrageously beneath his dignity, especially so when there are now so many Taiji dance instructors ready to flatter him and offer tea and biscuit instead of hard work when he attends their classes.

Question

Some styles, like Tai Chi and Dachengchuan, are rumored to be able to generate "empty force" to strike/bounce-off an opponent without actual' physically striking him/her.

What do you think of this ability?

Michael, Malaysia (August 1998)

Answer

It may be incredible, but such force is true. It is found in ma styles of kungfu besides Taijiquan and Dachengquan, and is k various names. In Shaolin Kungfu it is called pi-kong-zhang, or Across-Space Palm".

In classical times kungfu masters recognized "the three ulti "yi-the martial world", known in Chinese as "wu lin san jue". The Zen, zhi-chan", "pi-kong-zhang" and "shao-lin-shen-quan", or On three are Striking-across-Space Palm and Shaolin Marvelous Fist. A Shaolin arts.

Question

I have read your excellent book "The Complete Book of Tai Chi Chuan'" and am very interested in learning the Wudang Tai Chi form. From some things you said, I surmise that Wudang was devised as a non-traditional way of attaining health/longevity.

Also it seems good for self defense, especially compared with Wu or Yang styles, but without the elemental and very differentiated energies used in Chen.

Joss, United Kingdom (September 1999)

Answer

I do not know what you meant by non-traditional way of attaining health/longevity, but from the way I interpreted it, all the various styles of Taijiquan, including the Wudang Style, are traditional.

The Wudang Style is in fact the most traditional for attaining health and longevity as well as for attaining combat efficiency and spiritual fulfillment, and all other Taijiquan styles were derived from it.

By traditional, I meant following established traditions regarding both philosophy and practice. Some established traditions concerning the philosophy of Tai Chi Chuan include convictions that the aims of Tai Chi Chuan are to attain health, longevity, combat efficiency, and spiritual joy, and that the fundamental operating force to achieve these aims is chi.

Some established traditions concerning the practice of Taijiquan include showing respect to the master, training diligently every day, and emphasizing on developing "kung" rather than on learning techniques.

What, then, are the traditional ways of Tai Chi Chuan to attain health and longevity? They include employing appropriate movements, breathing and meditation to clear toxic waste, to increase energy volume and flow, to build a pearl of energy at the abdominal energy field, and to attain mental calmness and inner peace.

All styles of Tai Chi Chuan, if they are practiced as genuine Tai Chi Chuan, use these traditional ways. On the other hand, taking vitamins or jogging, running or skipping over a rope, and using mechanical means like hand weights are non-traditional.

In my opinion, much of Tai Chi taught today is non-traditional. Many Tai Chi practitioners or players are fond of saying that their art is internal, and they seldom have any experience of chi.

These are two glaring examples, although many people may be blind to the glare, that they have deviated from tradition. In other words, while Tai Chi Chuan is traditionally an internal, martial art, there is nothing internal or martial in much of the Tai Chi played today.

There is no doubt that all styles of Tai Chi Chuan are extremely good for self-defense. To say "it *seems* good" is insulting to Tai Chi Chuan masters, and a reflection on one's ignorance of Tai Chi Chuan as a great martial art.

Whether Wudang is more effective than Wu or Yang styles for self-defense depends on other factors, like how the students train and what the teachers teach, and not on the style itself.

I do not know what you meant by "elemental and very differentiated energies used in Chen". But energy or chi is elemental in all styles of Tai Chi Chuan. If different masters from the same or different styles use different terms to describe various applications of energy, it is for the convenience of understanding.

For example, Wudang and Chen Style masters often talk about "spiral force" used in executing a thrust punch. This form of energy application is also found in Yang Style and Wu Style, but is seldom mentioned because the thrust punch is seldom used.

Yang Style and Wu Style often mention "eight types of forces" which refer to the eight ways of applying energy in the eight fundamental Tai Chi Chuan techniques of their styles.

These "eight types of forces" are not mentioned in Wudang and Chen Style because these eight fundamental techniques were developed fror Chen Style, which itself did not specifically differentiate between t' eight techniques. Chen Style in turn was developed from Wudang Ta Chuan.

But this does not mean that Yang Style and Wu Style have techniques than Chen Style and Wudang, or that these eight types c are not found in Chen Style and Wudang.

In fact, Chen Style and Wudang have these techniques and energy application, but they were not specifically named.

Incidentally, this brings to mind that Chinese masters are ge an concerned with theoretical analysis, but with practical appli the opponent attacks them, what they are concern is successfully energy opponent a few feet backward; they are not bothered wheth an-jing they have used for the throw is called "qi-jing" (press-forc (push-force).

Then, why is there a differentiation into "qi-jing" and "an-jing"? This is for the sake of convenience. For example, after teaching a student how to develop and use energy in a certain way, he would say this is "qi-jing" so that the next time he mentions "qi-jing" the student would know what to do without the master having to repeat the process.

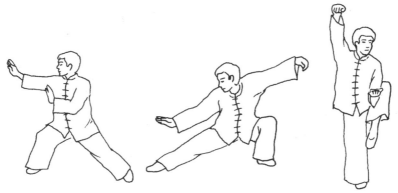

Chen Style Taijiquan   Yang Style Taijiquan   Wudang Style Taijiquan

Question

I practice Wudang Tai Chi. The lineage of my school is from Chen Tin-Hung in Hong Kong.
Peter, UK (July 1999)

Answer

If I am not mistaken, Sifu Chen Tin Hung of Hong Kong is the 4th generation successor of Sifu Wu Chuan You, the First Patriarch of Wu Style Taijiquan. Please note that in both Chinese writing and pronunciation, the "Chen" in the master's surname is different from the "Chen" in Chen 'tyle Taijiquan.

Although Sifu Chen Tin Hung is a Wu Style master, it was possible t he taught Wudang Taijiquan to some of his students, one of whom ht have passed on the Wudang set to later generations.

fu Chen is one of a very few masters who actively stressed Taijiquan irtial art. Besides being a sparring championship winner himself in ier days, he trained students who won numerous sparring ships in Hong Kong, Taiwan and South East Asia.

their ome pictures of this master taken in the 1970s. I am e-mailing in your files to you as souvenirs. Please feel free to pass them around l if you like.

Question

We have 24 yin-yang internal exercises as the basis of our system. I find these exercises very powerful — strengthening and energizing.

Recently a question has arisen over their origins.

I have received correspondence to the effect that these exercises came in fact from Hung Gar!

Peter, UK (July 1999)

Answer

As I have not seen how the exercises are performed, I would not be able to comment. Generally terms like "yin-yang internal exercises" are not usual in Hung Gar (Hoong Ka).

But the name could be misleading. It is possible that the exercises were originally named differently, but renamed with the term "yin-yang" to be more coherent with Taijiquan philosophy.

Question

But whether they have a common origin or which art has done the borrowing is something I am trying to find out. Given the fact that these exercises are inside the door teaching and are held to be the platform on which our tai chi is based this is a sensitive and difficult area.

I wonder if you or someone you know may be able to verify some things about them?

Peter, UK (July 1999)

Answer

Does it really matter whether it was Taijiquan that borrowed from Hung Gar, or Hung Gar that borrowed from Taijiquan, or that they had a common origin? After all, all great arts borrowed from one another. Shaolin Kung for example, borrowed much from Indian yoga and Taoist chi kung.

You will have more benefits, besides goodwill, if you spend your practicing the exercises instead of arguing over academic issues actually do not make much difference either way.

Hung Gar students are not likely to hug and kiss you even if y to prove that Taijiquan borrowed from Hung Gar. As these exe the "inside the door teaching" of your school, and have give presumably your classmates much benefit, your uncalled for would cause a lot of confusion and uncertainty.

On the other hand, proving that Hung Gar borrowed fro would not make you or your classmates better Taijiquan increase your practical benefits in any way. Hung Gar stude even bother to know the result of your discovery.

Question

We have 12 yin and 12 yang:

The 12 yin are: Golden turtle; Unity; Lifting a Golden Plate; Jade Rabbit Facing the Moon; Red Capped Crane Stretches its Feet; Civet Cat Catches Rats; Flicking the Whip on the Left and Right; White Ape Pushes Out its Paws; Swallow Pierces the Clouds; Leading A Goat Smoothly; Giant Python Turning its Body; and Elephant Shakes its Trunk.

All these are practiced in the horse riding stance.

This is interesting as our hand-form is closest to the Wu family hand-form which is the only style I know of to practice the Single Whip posture in the horse stance (as we do). The Wu family also has exercises in it very similar to these ones above.

Then the yang exercises are as follows: Golden Turtle; Tiger Paw; Dragon Coiled Round a Pillar; White Horse Pounds its Hooves; Planting a Fence; Wu Gang Cutting Laurels; and Rhinoceros Facing the Moon; etc.

Peter, UK (July 1999)

Answer

These are Wudang Taijiquan patterns, not Hung Gar patterns. The Horse-Riding Stance is used because the main purpose of these exercises is to develop internal force.

Question

I have been told that the 12 yin are the same as Da Mo's Yi Jin Jing (tendon changing classic).

Peter, UK (July 1999)

Answer

These "12 Yin" exercises and Bodhidharma's (Da Mo's) Yi Jin Jing re totally different. You have been misinformed.

stion

ould enlighten me at all? It is unfortunate is that there has been ion or misinformation in our teachings but if this is the case I feel y bound to find out and reveal the true state of affairs.

in urse I shall treat any information which you consider to be sensitive

Peter ost confidence.

July 1999)

Answer

You have made a rash conclusion. From the information provided by you, I think there has been no deception or misinformation in the teaching of your school.

Even if we suppose that what your school claimed to be from Taijiquan were taken from Hung Gar, it was at its worst misinformation; we cannot call it deception as there was no malicious intention to cheat you.

Let us take our supposition a step further. Suppose there was an intention to deceive you. In other words, let us suppose your teacher knew the exercises were originally from Hung Gar, but he wittingly told you they were from Taijiquan.

Even using this supposition, there is no need for you to create a storm in a teacup to embarrass your teacher and your school, especially when he has so kindly given you his "inside the door teaching" that has made you powerful and energetic. You are lucky: you have a chance to develop internal force in your Taijiquan class; a great majority of Taiji students merely learn to dance.

In kungfu culture, there are other values besides being duty bound and being truthful, such as honoring the master, being grateful and being generous. In your case, you have confused being duty bound and being truthful with bravado and pettiness.

You should clean up your own room before attempting to clean up the whole house. In other words, you should correct your own faults before attempting to correct the faults of others.

If you, for example, look at your paragraph above (left unedited for this purpose), you will notice a number of spelling and grammatical errors, which indicate both carelessness and mediocrity.

Common sense can tell us that if one cannot even write a letter wel¹ is unlikely he has the capability to correct a widespread practice or co affecting many people.

Please do not mistake my well-intended comments as severe cr I am offering a fresh perspective which I am sure will not only improve your martial art training but also to enhance your daily ' play.

Question

My teacher primarily taught the Lee family style of Tai·ˢ· which I have found to be almost unknown amongst other pr

Is it known to you?

Tom, UK (September 1999)

Answer

I have heard of the Lee style, but I do not know much about it. Through the years, Tai Chi Chuan masters, generally of the Yang style originally, have sometimes used their own surnames to describe their styles, but these styles are usually known only within their own circles. The Lee style is probably one of them.

Question

I would like to know more about the nature of internal force, relative to external strength generated by muscles. For example, I read somewhere that the late Taijiquan master Cheng Man Ch'ing was able to throw someone across a room, yet he was unable to lift a bowling ball.

On the other hand, I believe you mentioned in one of your question and answer series that the Eighteen Lohan Hands and related techniques in Shaolin Kungfu increased the physical strength of the exponent.
Chia-Hua, USA (October 1999)

Answer

In kungfu and chi kung, terms are often used provisionally, i.e. they are used for the convenient understanding of the situation in question. Unlike scientific terms, they are not used to define (which actually means to limit) items or events exclusively.

In other words, in an orthodox scientific context, if "internal force" is A, it cannot be B; but in a kungfu or chi kung context, "internal force" can be A in one situation, and B in another situation. This in fact is also the everyday context. For example, you may regard Mary pretty in one situation, but selfish in another situation.

The term "internal force" is used provisionally to distinguish it from "external strength". Generally, internal force refers to force (or ability to do work) that is generated inside the body, particularly by energy flow and mind. External strength refers to strength, or force, that is generated by muscles which are considered relatively outside the body.

Of course, someone who wishes to split hair, or who wants to be ific, can argue that energy flow and mind can be outside the body, scles can be inside the body.

fu and chi kung masters are not interested in such arguments; un more interested in using the two terms provisionally for better ing and better performances.

Sifu Cheng Man Ching could throw someone across a room but presumably could not lift a bowling ball in his old age because the kind of force used were different in the two situations.

Sifu Cheng was an undisputed master in applying his internal force to throw people, as this was important in Taijiquan (for combat, for example); but lifting a bowling ball was not important and hence he did not want to waste his time training himself to do that.

On the other hand, an Eagle Claw master can apply his internal force to lift a bowling ball many times heavier, but he may be unable to throw a person like what Sifu Cheng did. The reason is the same. Gripping an opponent is important in Eagle Claw Kungfu, and he must grip a lot of heavy objects in his training; but throwing a person across a room is not important to him.

Hence, in their training, the Eagle Claw master focuses on channeling his internal force to his fingers, whereas Sifu Cheng focused on exploding his internal force out of his palms.

I was told that in his old age, the Aikido grandmaster Uyeshiba was too weak to walk, and had to be carried by his disciples to the training hall to see students practice. But when the old grandmaster demonstrated his skills, he could easily throw able bodied people a third his age and three times his weight!

All genuine Shaolin arts develop the exponent holistically, i.e. developing his physical body as well as his energy and mind. In practicing the Eighteen Lohan Hands or various Shaolin Kungfu techniques, the exponent, besides other benefits, loosens and strengthens his muscles and joints, thus adding to his physical strength.

A major problem with many Shaolin students today is that they only pay attention to the physical aspects, without realizing the more important aspects of energy and mind.

Question

Dear Wong Sifu,

I would like to know how would Tai Chi Chuan fair against other martial arts in combat.

I am aware about some of the wonderful benefits practicing Tai Chi Chuan can bring to your life, like heightened awareness, grace, improved health, activeness even in old age, self-defense without the compromise of deterioration of the body, character development, and even spiritual discoveries in advanced stages.

However, with all other multitudinous plus points aside, how useful is Tai Chi Chuan in combat against other martial arts?

Hui, Singapore (August 1999)

Answer

Tai Chi Chuan is basically a martial art. All the benefits you have mentioned about Tai Chi Chuan are true, yet they are only secondary benefits which Tai Chi Chuan exponents get as a bonus; the primary benefit of Tai Chi Chuan is combat efficiency which is a logical result of the primary aim of Tai Chi Chuan as a martial art.

In other words, in the past people practiced Tai Chi Chuan not because they wanted to have heightened awareness, grace, improved health, etc., but because they wanted to fight well. Heightened awareness, grace, improved health, etc. came about as a bonus of practicing Tai Chi Chuan for combat. Even the bonus is so wonderful; this will give an idea how more wonderful is the main result, i.e. its effectiveness for combat.

Theoretically speaking, considering combative factors like force, techniques and strategies, Tai Chi Chuan is far superior in combat than many martial arts or martial sports like Judo, Aikido, Karate, Taekwondo, Western Boxing and even Siamese Boxing.

One crucial point that many people often do not realize is that these other arts are sports, governed by safety rules, whereas Tai Chi Chuan is not limited by any rules. In a real fight in the past if these martial artists were to use their typical techniques to attack a Tai Chi Chuan master, they would be killed or seriously injured.

For example, if a Judo exponent were to hold a Tai Chi Chuan master to prepare for a throw, the master could kill the Judo exponent with a devastating palm strike on the head.

If a Taekwondo exponent were to use high kicks to attack the Tai Chi Chuan master, the master can easily counter the attack by attacking the opponent's groin.

Such a situation does not happen today because of two reasons.

One, ours is a law-abiding society; real fights in the past where killing or maiming was common, are happily obsolete.

Two, very, very few people today practice Tai Chi Chuan; most people perform Tai Chi dance, and of course Tai Chi dance is no match for these martial arts or sports.

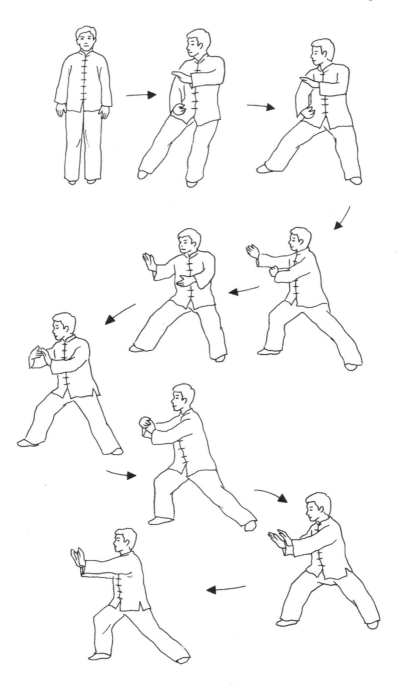

Grasping Sparrow's Tail

Question

My acquaintance told me that all kungfu (as well as Tai Chi Chuan) is useless against modern combative arts like Brazilian Jujutsu, Vale Tudo, and especially Muai Thai.

I also received a URL from him on his page that supposedly showed that all kungfu inferior to these "formless" martial arts (this term was popularized after Bruce Lee said that kungfu emphasized too much on "classical forms" and "dead techniques", and that his fighting was formless).

Hui, Singapore (August 1999)

Answer

Your acquaintance did not have a chance to know real kungfu, including Tai Chi Chuan. This is in fact the norm. Very, very few people have the chance to experience real kungfu; most people practice or witness kungfu gymnastics or dance.

How many kungfu students you know, for example, spend time on force training and methodical sparring, which are crucial aspects of real kungfu?

Most of them spend most of, if not all, their time on form practice, which is in many ways the least important aspect of kungfu. Those who have spent all their lives demonstrating forms to please spectators, and have never learnt to spar at all, will be no match against any fighter.

The forms in kungfu are the crystallization of centuries of real fighting techniques. In the beginning people fought without forms. Then they discovered that by adopting certain positions and using certain movements in given combat situations, they would have certain advantages.

For example, instead of punching in a haphazard manner with their feet apart, they found that they would have more power as well as stability if they placed one leg in front of the other and punched from their waist, spiraling the fist in the punching momentum.

This gradually developed into the technique of thrusting a punch at the bow-arrow stance. This technique, executed in this way, constitutes a kungfu pattern, and is named in Shaolin Kungfu as "Black Tiger Steals Heart".

When a fighter using the "Black Tiger Steal Heart" pattern was counter-attacked by an opponent using a side kick, he could respond in numerous ways. Masters discovered that one good way was merely shifting the body backward, without moving the feet, as this would give the exponent speed as well as conversion of energy. This developed into the pattern called "Taming a Tiger with a String of Beads".

Later the masters discovered that instead of merely avoiding the kick, the exponent could strike the kicking leg, thus gaining the advantage of striking an opponent at a time when his initial attack is just spent. This developed into the pattern "Lohan Strikes Drum".

These two patterns underwent further development in Tai Chi Chuan. In line with "softness" in Tai Chi Chuan, the Shaolin "Black Tiger" pattern evolved into the softer Tai Chi pattern called "Punch Below Sleeves", where energy flow instead of speed and momentum is emphasized.

Instead of striking the opponent's leg using the comparatively forceful "Lohan Strikes Drum", a Tai Chi Chuan exponent would use the softer "lu" technique of "Grasping Sparrow's Tail" to grip and dislocate the opponent's ankle.

These kungfu techniques, manifested in kungfu patterns, were not invented by someone sitting in an ivory tower, but were evolved through actual fighting over many centuries.

To untrained persons, these techniques would be cumbersome; it would be easier and more "natural" for them to throw a punch in an ordinary standing position or to jump away when kicked at, than to use the Black Tiger or the Lohan patterns.

One needs to spend a lot of time to practice these patterns until they become second nature, and even more time to practice to enable one to use these patterns effectively in combat.

Most kungfu students lack the method or the patience for such practice. As a result, even though they may perform these patterns beautifully in solo demonstrations, they are unable to use them at all in combat.

Despite what Bruce Lee said, he used forms in his fighting. He did not kick haphazardly, he adopted certain positions and kicked in certain ways so as to have definite combative advantages, particularly power and speed. His forms, nevertheless, resemble more of Taekwondo than of traditional kungfu.

What Bruce Lee meant was one should not be slavishly tied to his forms. More significantly he emphasized that kungfu forms were for fighting, not for beautiful demonstrations.

He was remembered for echoing the kungfu tenet, "kungfu progresses from formless to form, then completing the full circle from form to formless". In other words, before one learns kungfu, he fights haphazardly.

Then he learns kungfu forms, which gives him the most advantageous techniques for fighting. Having mastered the forms, he may modify them to suit the particular combat situations.

There is no doubt that Bruce Lee was a great fighter, and he contributed much to the popularity of kungfu. But, paradoxically, I think his understanding of traditional kungfu was not deep.

I must clarify that I am merely stating my opinion, and I mean no disrespect to this great fighter.

Had his understanding of kungfu been deep, he would have used traditional kungfu techniques in combat instead of those of Taekwondo; he would have used traditional kungfu force training involving mind and energy instead of using western mechanical means; and most crucially he would have realized the importance of gradual progress and not have over trained and abused himself.

Yet, having said all these, we salute this man who gave his life to martial arts.

Question

The site had examples of kungfu, Tai Chi Chuan, and san shou exponents losing to Muai Thai exponents.

In fact, according to him, history has proved so far (in the fights) that kungfu cannot handle the moves in other "formless" martial arts.

According to my acquaintance, nobody ever attacked Tai Chi experts of the past like Yang Lu Chan with low roundhouse kicks to the thighs "that will make one unable to even stand" or "grab his neck/head and throw continuous knees into his ribs."

Hence, he concluded that Tai Chi experts are no match to "formless" fighting, and is an obsolete art for combat.

Hui, Singapore (August 1999)

Answer

Your acquaintance based his conclusion on the shameful performances of kungfu gymnasts and Tai Chi dancers, most of whom have never sparred in their lives, and his knowledge of kungfu history is grossly limited.

Obviously he did not know that in the late 19th and early 20th centuries, many martial art masters from many foreign countries went to China to test the Chinese masters, and virtually all of them were defeated.

For those used to thinking Tai Chi dance is Tai Chi Chuan, it is difficult to imagine how extremely powerful and combat efficient Tai Chi Chuan masters like Yang Lu Chan were.

Yang Lu Chan went round China to test his own skills, meeting masters of various styles, and he was never defeated, earning the nickname "Yang the Ever Victorious".

Some masters would have used the low roundhouse kicks, known in kungfu as "whirlwind kicks" on him, and he could easily counter with an appropriate modification of his favorite Tai Chi pattern "Grasping Sparrow's Tail", throwing the attackers to the ground.

No one would be so foolish as to try grabbing his neck or head, or throwing continuous knees into his ribs, for that would be asking for trouble. With the opponent in such unguarded close quarters, all Yang Lu Chan had to do was to strike his powerful Tai Chi palm into the opponent's chest, killing or seriously injuring him.

Please refer to the article titled **What could a Taijiquan master like Yang Lu Chan do if a Muai Thai fighter grabs his neck or head and throws continuous knees into his ribs?** on my web-site for some details on Taijiquan techniques against Muai Thai knee jabs.

My hometown, Sungai Petani, is near Thailand, the home of Muai Thai. Some of my students were Muai Thai fighters and instructors before they learnt Shaolin Kungfu from me.

My Shaolin students could handle ferocious Muai Thai techniques from these fighters quite comfortably. I owed this to my master, Sifu Ho Fatt Nam, who was a professional, not just an amateur, Muai Thai fighter and champion before he gave it up for Shaolin Kungfu. My students and I are no where when compared with Yang Lu Chan; this is not modesty, I am being honest.

Remember also that happily in our modern days, sparring — even amongst professionals — is taken as a sport. But in the past in China, combat was often a serious life-death matter. Combatants fully knew that a slight mistake or a poor defense might cost them their lives.

They simply had to be good fighters to survive. This will give an idea of the difference in standard between real combat in the past and sparring today, even with ferocious Muai Thai fighters.

You may explain to your acquaintance to help him widen his perspective, but if he insists that formless martial art or Muai Thai is superior, there is no necessity to argue with him. His narrow-mindedness constitutes his loss, not yours.

If we are convinced that Shaolin Kungfu or Tai Chi Chuan is a great martial art, we practice diligently to derive the benefits, and perhaps share it with those who sincerely seek our help. But we have no need to prove to others, or to waste time arguing with those who stubbornly close their mind.

Question

What troubles me is that what I trust to be a great, advanced art that is perfected over the ages can actually be beaten by someone who spends (significantly) less time on a newly created martial art.

Aren't Shaolin Kungfu and Tai Chi Chuan widely known to be the best fighting arts in the world? Can you enlighten me on this?

Hui, Singapore (August 1999)

Answer

Shaolin Kungfu and Tai Chi Chuan are the greatest martial arts in the world, and their greatness lies beyond fighting. When I was still a boy I read a master saying that comparing other martial arts with Chinese martial arts is like comparing a drop of water with an ocean.

At that time I thought he was chauvinistic and exaggerating beyond reasons. But now, having experienced the scope and depth of Shaolin Kungfu and Tai Chi Chuan, I am beginning to see the truth in his comparison.

You are disappointed because you, like most people, have mistaken external demonstrative forms, known as "flowery fists and embroidery kicks" in idiomatic Chinese, for real kungfu.

The fact is that real kungfu, whether Shaolin or Tai Chi Chuan, is very, very rare; what we normally see is external demonstrative forms. Because of its scope and depth, it is understandable that we need much more time to be proficient in real kungfu, but once we are properly and sufficiently trained, defending ourselves against opponents of other martial arts would not be a problem.

Question

At the same time, it also puzzles me. The ultimate combat goal of all "internal" martial arts especially is to become formless.

How is it that such famous kungfu experts are still fighting in forms? Or is real kungfu and Tai Chi Chuan really inferior to these new arts?

Hui, Singapore (August 1999)

Answer

The expression that at an advanced stage Chinese martial artists (not just the internal ones) become formless in combat, means that the decisive factor in combat has shifted from techniques (which have form) to force (which is formless).

If you have so much internal force, it does not matter what forms or techniques you use, just one strike on your opponent is enough to finish him off.

This will also give you an idea of the different standard between Chinese martial arts and the other arts.

A Karate punch or a Taekwondo kick may be destructive when connected on an untrained person, but to a Chinese master with Golden Bell, Iron Shirt or other forms of internal force, the punch or kick actually does not worry him much. But just one strike of his Iron Palm, Cosmos Palm or an attack packed by tremendous internal force may kill or maim.

This is one reason why freely kicking and punching each other in sparring which is normal in many other martial arts, is unthinkable in kungfu.

In another dimension, formlessness refers to mind, in contrast to physical body. Have you heard of this expression, which is not commonly mentioned: "In advanced kungfu you fight with your heart"? Here "heart" means mind, and is formless.

At the highest level, formlessness refers to the greatest spiritual achievement. In Shaolin Kungfu it is attaining Zen or enlightenment; in Tai Chi Chuan it is attaining Tao or returning to the Great Void.

Question

How would Tai Chi Chuan fair against Chinese martial arts with confusing and strange footwork like Baguazhang and Drunken Fist, or Monkey Kungfu? Tai Chi Chuan, like Chang Chuan, seems very direct and straight forward.

Would this not be a disadvantage against such styles with confusing and unpredictable footwork?

Hui, Singapore (August 1999)

Answer

In terms of combat efficiency, Tai Chi Chuan, Baguazhang, Drunken Fist and Monkey Kungfu belong to the same very high level of kungfu.

In terms of mind expansion and spiritual cultivation, Tai Chi Chuan is the highest, Baguazhang next, whereas Drunken Fist and Monkey Kungfu are basically meant for fighting.

Because of historical development, different needs and other reasons, they have different emphasis in their approach to combat. Tai Chi Chuan makes much use of circular movements and energy flow, whereas the other three emphasize on agile footwork.

While Tai Chi Chuan and Baguazhang are comparatively more straight-forward, Drunken Fist and Monkey Kungfu make use of deceptive moves. All these four styles use internal force.

If all other things are equal, then these styles with confusing and unpredictable footwork would be an advantage over Tai Chi Chuan. But other things are not equal.

Although in comparison a Tai Chi Chuan exponent generally remains at his stance, his circular movements make him very versatile.

So instead of moving his feet in agile footwork to avoid an attack, he merely swerves his body to deflect the attacking force, then turning it back to the opponent, thus securing an advantage instead of a disadvantage.

Thus whether a Tai Chi Chuan exponent is a better fighter than one practicing Baguazhang, Drunken Fist or Monkey Kungfu will depend on numerous formless variables like force, skill and temperament, besides the form variables of techniques.

Question
I read in a Baguazhang book that Xing Yi is good for close range, Tai Chi Chuan is good for middle and close ranges, while Baguazhang is good for all ranges.

Does this mean that Baguazhang is superior to Tai Chi Chuan, since it can handle attacks of all ranges, or is this an insignificant piece of information when it comes to actual self-defense?
Hui, Singapore (August 1999)

Answer
I disagree with the opinion mentioned in that book. To me, all these three arts are good for all ranges.

If Baguazhang or Xing Yi Kungfu were superior to Tai Chi Chuan, then more people would practice these two arts. But in fact the number of Tai Chi Chuan exponents far outnumber that of Baguazhang or Xing Yi Kungfu.

While the number of exponents itself is not a definite indication of the superiority of an art as other factors are also involved, it does has some relationship.

Question
No matter what your answer is, I will still practice my Tai Chi Chuan with diligence and hard-work to bring myself to a good level of combat efficiency and where I will fully benefit from the art, because Tai Chi Chuan is a great part of my culture.
Hui, Singapore (August 1999)

Answer

While you attitude reveals that you are proud of your cultural roots, it may not necessarily be a wise one.

If, for example, my answer were very unfavorable to Tai Chi Chuan — which of course it was not — you should seek a second, and then a third opinion.

If all expert opinions expressed that Tai Chi Chuan were an inferior art, you should have the courage to accept the inferiority of your roots and change to a better art, or if you have the capabilities, improve it. But as it is, Tai Chi Chuan is a wonderful art.

What is important is that you should differentiate between Tai Chi dance and Tai Chi Chuan.

If you continue practicing Tai Chi dance you will further the degradation of a wonderful art, bring shame and ridicule to it like what your acquaintance had done. But practicing real Tai Chi Chuan is not easy as it is very difficult to find a genuine Tai Chi Chuan master, and even if you have found one, it is very demanding to practice it.

The rewards, however, are worth the time and effort.

Question

I have come to Tai Chi Chuan reasonably late in life as a result of seeking relief from painful sciatica.

Over the past two years the sciatica has, dare I say, disappeared, my weight has reduced, vitality increased and I have regained the spirit of the searcher that I had some years ago.

Jon, UK (October 1999)

Answer

This is wonderful. Carry on with your practice.

Training

Question

You told me that if my practice of an hour a day is appropriate I should reach a good standard within a year.

I am sorry if this is a rather inevitable question but I would be most appreciative if you would point me in the right direction as to what is appropriate.

Richard, UK (July 1998)

Answer

What is appropriate in your practice (about an hour a day) so that you can attain a fairly high level in a year, depends on numerous factors like you aims and objectives, your needs and abilities as well as available instructions and supportive material.

Presuming that your aim is to learn genuine Taijiquan (and not Taiji dance), that you are willing to put in some time and effort, and that you have difficulty finding a good master in your area but you have my "The Complete Book of Tai Chi Chuan" as supportive material, I would suggest the following training program.

The time frames are suggestions and in most cases may run concurrently. For example, you need not wait for one month and two hours before starting "Lifting Water"; you can start immediately or perhaps two weeks later.

1. Read "The Complete Book of Tai Chi Chuan" and other Taijiquan books if available, to have a sound understanding of the philosophy, scope and depth of Taijiquan. This should take about a month.

2. Define your aims and objectives. You may, for example, aim to find out whether you can experience the wonderful benefits of Taijiquan by following my suggestions, and your objectives may include experiencing some internal force through the "Lifting Water" exercise, and attaining balance and relaxation through various Taijiquan movements for two hours.

3. Practice "Lifting Water" for six months. Refer to my book for details.

4. Practice the Wuji Stance after "Lifting Water" for six months.

5. Practice the fundamental Taijiquan movements described in chapter 5 of my book — three months. Begin this stage only after at least one month of "Lifting Water" and "Wuji Stance". Seek an instructor to get your movements smooth and proper. Even if the instructor teaches Taiji dance instead of Taijiquan, you can still benefit a lot from him regarding the Taijiquan movements. It is all right if the movements he teaches are different form the ones I describe in my book.

6. Learn and practice the 24-Pattern Taijiquan Simplified Set (described in Chapter 7 of my book) or any suitable Taijiquan set from a master if you are lucky enough to find one, or from a Taiji dance instructor for 4 months. Learn this or any other Taijiquan sets only after you have spent some time over the fundamental Taijiquan movements in stage 5.

7. Continue to practice the Taijiquan set but with focus on energy flow and mind for 4 months. Please refer to my book for guidance.

8. Find yourself a partner to practice "Pushing Hands" for 3 months. If you cannot find a partner, imagine you have one.
9. Find a real or imaginary partner to practice combat application of Taijiquan for 4 months.

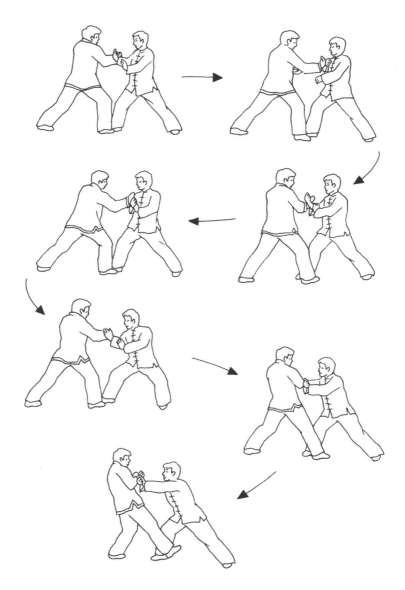

Pushing Hands Exercise

Question

From what you have written, it would seem my best approach might be to do something like the following

1. Practice one or two dynamic Chi Kung exercises, as well as doing some self-manifested movements, to help develop internal energy
2. Extend into abdominal breathing practice under the guidance of a master ONLY after having done the Chi Kung exercises for some months
3. Practice doing one or two of the Tai Chi postures and 'getting them right'
4. Practice one or two of the 13 techniques, 'getting them right'

Is this what you were suggesting? Have I understood you correctly?

Richard, UK (July 1998)

Answer

Yes, but this is only the start.

You have to get into the Taijiquan techniques too. One good way is to learn and practice a typical Taijiquan set well. At the same time you continue with your force or skill training.

When you are familiar with the Taijiquan techniques, and have sufficient skills, proceed to combat application. You should also ensure that your Taijiquan training will enrich your daily life, such as mental clarity and vitality in your work and play.

Question

You mentioned in your book "The Complete Book of Tai Chi Chuan" that Chen Style is famous for its martial aspects.

However, I also hear that it takes very long to be good in Tai Chi self-defense (about 10 years?).

This is very discouraging for me since that is the main aim of my Tai Chi Chuan.

Xavier, Singapore (September 1999)

Answer

If you have a good teacher and you are willing to work hard, you should be able to handle a black-belt within two years, irrespective of which style of kungfu (including Chen Style Tai Chi Chuan) you practice.

While Tai Chi Chuan is very effective for self-defense, that is not its greatest benefit. If, for some reason, your sole purpose is self-defense, you would achieve your purpose better by choosing a waijia (external style) kungfu.

But making self-defense your only aim in practicing kungfu is not a wise choice.

Question

I have been practicing Yang Style Taijiquan for about 2 years. I am sometimes called upon by small groups and individuals to demonstrate the Beijing short form, Yang main form and some Qiqong forms for the purposes of relaxation.

This I do without hesitation for although I have not practiced for long enough to call myself a teacher, I do feel that by being in a situation where others can follow my movements and gain benefit from them, then I am doing somebody, myself included, a little bit of good.
Paul, United Kingdom (December 1998)

Answer

Without knowing it, you are doing them a great disservice — you are encouraging them to practice Taiji dance instead of Taijiquan.

You can read about the difference between Taiji dance, which most people do today, and Taijiquan, done by great masters in the past, in my home page on Taijiquan.

Question

I have been practicing Tai Chi for the past 7 months at 30 minutes per day.

I would like to focus my taiji to the level that I can use my chi to heal my relatives of common ailments like stomach aches or muscle spasms.

Please instruct me which of your books is the most suitable for this matter.
Tim, USA (September 1999)

Answer

You attitude towards Tai Chi Chuan and other eastern arts is quite common among many people in the West.

There is no question about your and the other people's sincerity in wanting to help others, but obviously you have a grossly mistaken concept of both the philosophy as well as the practice of these arts.

Let us take Tai Chi Chuan as an example. As Tai Chi Chuan is a martial art, the primary purpose of practicing it, is — or was, according to all its masters, before it has been so ridiculously diluted — combat efficiency.

It has never been the intention of real Tai Chi Chuan masters to train their students to be healers.

Nevertheless, some real Tai Chi Chuan masters and advanced exponents do have the ability to use their chi, or vital energy, to help friends and relatives recover from ailments like stomach aches and muscle spasms.

The reason is actually simple. At the most fundamental level, all ailments are caused by energy blockage, and because the energy flow of the masters and advanced exponents is so powerful, it can help to clear the blockage. But this ability to overcome ailments with their chi is a bonus, not the focus of their Tai Chi Chuan training.

It is really amazing that so many people in the West think that such advanced skills of energy management, including developing one's vital energy and using it to help others, can be readily learnt from reading a book or viewing a video.

Sometimes I receive e-mails from people who have no chi kung experience before, but asking me to describe chi kung exercises to them so that they can teach their friends to overcome cancer! It is as ridiculous as asking a surgeon to recommend his favorite text book so that they can read up on surgery and then operate on their friends.

It is commendable that you wish to develop your chi so that eventually you may help others. But you have to bear in mind three things.

One, you must learn personally from a master.

Two you must be willing to put in a lot of time and effort in your training.

Three, you have to make sure you yourself is healthy and full of vitality before you think of healing others.

Incidentally, the third point is not frequently observed in the West. Many of the healers, usually self-trained, I have met in the West are themselves suffering from pains and illnesses.

Question

Can you point me toward any info on the Taiji sword forms?

I am currently learning the first of these and would like some help in knowing what and where to purchase my prize for finishing my form, that is a proper sword for demonstration purposes.

Paul, United Kingdom ((December 1998)

Answer

I would sincerely suggest for your benefit that you should postpone learning your Taiji sword dance, and concentrate on finding a master to practice genuine Taijiquan.

Only when you can generate chi, or intrinsic energy, to your hands should you consider learning the Taijiquan sword.

You will find much information on Taijiquan, including the Taijiquan sword, in my book, "The Complete Book of Tai Chi Chuan".

Question

Sifu, I have started learning Taiji.

We went to 5 schools that offered it but after seeing their interpretation of the Lohan pattern (extremely karate-like) we decided to learn from videos.

I know it sounds vain but we decided to learn by ourselves first so we could properly tell what to look for in an instructor.

Ron, USA (December 1998)

Answer

The Lohan set is not found in Taijiquan. It could be added by someone who did not fully understand Taijiquan or Lohanquan (Lohan Kungfu).

If you examine the issue historically, it was precisely because the great Zhang San Feng found Shaolin Lohanquan not ideal for his purpose that he modified it, which led to the development of Taijiquan.

Others, whose purpose and situation are different from Zhang San Feng's, may find Lohanquan more suitable. One should, therefore, practice Taijiquan or Lohanquan, or any martial art (not necessarily Chinese kung fu) which is ideal for his purpose.

Genuine Taijiquan and Lohanquan are complete arts themselves; they do not need to incorporate anything from outside. And good Taijiquan or Lohanquan is never karate-like.

One who introduces Lohanquan into Taijiquan, or vice versa, is an example of what the Chinese proverb says as "knowing the surface but not knowing the inside".

Because of his limited knowledge (although this limited knowledge may be much, when compared with what his students and the general public know) he honestly thinks he is doing his art and his students a great service, when actually he is doing a great disservice, because without his knowing he is hindering the potential development of his students (although his students may have some little gains initially), and he is debasing his art, undoing the many centuries of development past masters have accumulated.

The above explanation applies to those practicing genuine Taijiquan or Lohanquan. If one is doing Taiji dance or Lohan dance, which is actually the norm today, adding something from one art to the other is generally beneficial.

Further, the explanation applies to arts, like Taijiquan and Lohanquan, that have already reached a very, very high level of development. In the case of a low level art, incorporating something useful into it is generally good. A very rough analogy is as follows.

If you can speak Chinese very well, you need not worry about putting English grammar into your Chinese, or vice versa. But if you hardly knew Chinese or English, mixing the two languages together might sometimes serve your purpose better.

In your particular case, learning some Taijiquan (but not Lohanquan) may be useful. This of course does not imply that Tsoi Li Hoi Kungfu or its parental Choy-Li-Fatt Kungfu is a low level art.

In fact, Choy-Li-Fatt is highly developed, and is one of the most famous martial arts in the world today. It was modified from Shaolin Kungfu by by the great masters Chen Harng and Cheong Hoong Sing for a particular purpose — combat efficiency, especially fighting en mass in revolutionary warfare.

If one's aim is combat efficiency, which in fact is why one practices kungfu, Choy-Li-Fatt is an excellent choice. But if you wish to go beyond combat efficiency, such as internal force training and spiritual cultivation, Choy-Li-Fatt and many other kungfu styles by themselves may be inadequate.

This is because the early Choy-Li-Fat masters, in their revolutionary situations, did not pay much attention to such dimensions as these did not serve their purpose well, and their decisions, thoughts and practice have set a definite direction for the development of their art.

The energy flow and meditative aspects of genuine Taijiquan will provide where Choy-Li-Fatt may lack. I must mention that this is not a slight on Choy-Li-Fatt Kungfu. In other aspects, such as stretching muscles and improving agility, Choy-Li-Fatt may be better than Taijiquan. But you must practice genuine Taijiquan where energy flow and meditation are integral features.

If you merely do Taiji dance, you would probably waste your time because your own kungfu style can provide you with agility, balance, gracefulness and stamina more effectively than Taiji dance can provide.

Alternatively you can practice genuine Shaolin Kungfu instead of Taijiquan for your purpose. Personally, all other things being equal, I think this is a better approach because both the philosophy and practice of Shaolin Kungfu are more conducive to Choy-Li-Fatt Kungfu.

Choy-Li-Fatt was evolved from Shaolin Kungfu, which originally had (and still have) all the internal aspects. Choy-Li-Fatt masters did not make use of these internal aspects not because they were not there but because they were not needed.

Now, when situations have changed, you may want to go back to your source and make good use of the treasure which was originally there.

It is a good idea to learn from video for your mentioned purpose, so long as you remember that unless one is already familiar with the art, learning from video only gives him the outward form, which is in many ways the least important aspect of the art.

The more important aspects of Taijiquan and Lohanquan as well as other kungfu styles are the energy and the mind aspects, if we view kungfu from the perspectives of form, energy and mind.

If we view it from the perspectives of form, force, application and philosophy, the more important aspects are force and application.

In other words, one's kungfu form may be beautiful or his philosophy convincing, but if he does not have kungfu force or is unable to apply what he has learnt in combat and his daily life, all his form and philosophy are useless.

Question

I was wondering about your thoughts on weight training and if it is counter-productive to the principals of Tai Chi.

I would really like to restart a weight training regimen, but have read several articles that have been negative with regards to Tai Chi.
Cyrus, USA (January 1999)

Answer

I fully agree with the view held by virtually all past masters that weight training is counter-productive to the principles of Tai Chi Chuan.

The reason is quite simple, although it may not be apparent to most westerners who generally think that power can only be built through muscles.

Weight training works on muscles, which is physical, whereas the force of Taijiquan is derived from energy flow, which is internal. Tensing muscles which is quite inevitable in weight training constricts energy flow, which is therefore detrimental to Taijiquan force development.

I would strongly advise against a weight training regimen.

Even if you leave aside Taijiquan force development, but look at middle aged people who had weight training in their younger days, it is not uncommon to find many of them weak and sickly.

On the other hand, those who develop their force through energy flow, in Taijiquan or other arts, are still fit and healthy at eighty.

Question

I have started practicing Yang style Taijiquan and I was wondering if it would be possible to combine the stance training and the first form training with my chi kung training.
Pushpinder (June 1998)

Answer

Taijiquan itself is a form of chi kung. Indeed, without the training of chi, it ceases to be Taijiquan and often degenerates into Taiji dance.

For various reasons, more than 90% of people who think they practice Taijiquan are actually doing Taiji dance. Practicing Taiji dance is not without its benefits.

It promotes grace and balance, as well as improves blood circulation, but it does not give the benefits that Taijiquan is well known to give, such as being fit and healthy at 60 and beyond, mentally fresh, combat efficient and having internal force.

Chi kung means "energy work". If you work on your energy, such as consciously generating energy flow, when practicing Taijiquan, you are already doing chi kung.

If you merely work on your muscles or body form, such as paying attention to where you should place your hands and feet, you are merely doing Taijiquan form which virtually all Taijiquan masters and classics have said is the least important.

You can also combine or supplement your Taijiquan practice with other forms of chi kung training. You can, for example, perform "Lifting the Sky" or "Carrying the Moon" or any dynamic patterns from any chi kung styles before starting your Taijiquan set, and conclude the set with standing or, if you are advanced, sitting meditation.

Question

I met a tai chi sifu here and he showed me some movements that I tried but it was too painful to do them so I stopped. I would like to improve my flexibility but as I said before I cannot warm up.

Do you know a way to stretch without warming up so I would not hurt myself?

William, Sweden (October 1997)

Answer

From the western perspective, one has to warm up before doing stretching exercises.

Hence you have a problem: you want to improve your flexibility but you can not warm up.

However, this is a problem only if you view it from a typical western perspective.

From the chi kung or kungfu perspective, the problem is irrelevant, because one can achieve flexibility without first having to warm up.

This may sound odd to someone used to the western way of thinking about warming up and stretching. But if you take a few minutes to reflect, you may even find this western view odd.

For example, if someone were to attack you, you do not ask your attacker to wait while you warm up; you have to react immediately, and you have to be flexible in your reaction in order to handle the attacker effectively.

A kungfu student is trained to handle attacks immediately and effectively. Many of the chi kung exercises explained in my books can enable you to be flexible without the necessity of warming up in the western manner.

Question

As regards class development, should the Taijiquan instructors emphasize relaxation?

They say they do not remember that you taught them how to relax in the Taijiquan courses.

Adalia, Spain (October 2000)

Answer

Relaxation is of utmost importance in Taijiquan and all internal arts.

If one cannot relax, he (or she) cannot manage internal force. In the Taijiquan courses (in Segovia, Spain in August) I taught everyone to relax, not just once or twice, but all the time, and everyone did well.

If they had not relaxed, they would not have the results that they had, such as having remarkable internal force, and feeling joyful and peaceful inside — results which many of them reported to the class during discussion.

The way I taught them relaxation was different from what they might have imagined. That is why they might not remember my teaching them relaxation.

I did not, for example, say, "Listen, you are going to learn relaxation. First you have to do this, then this, and this and this." This is textbook teaching, what many Taiji readers (in contrast to practitioners) might expect.

My teaching was informal. By various subtle ways I got the students to relax, even before they realized it.

Later they could relax on their own, with little or no help from me. Only when they were relaxed and focused, could they proceed to other Taijiquan skills.

This is an example of transmission of skills, which is qualitatively different from listing of techniques.

Do you remember the time we did combat application where even small sized women could throw big sized men to the ground.

If the women were not relaxed they could not have done that — had they tensed their muscles in their throws, the women would not have sufficient physical strength to throw hefty men.

I recall one woman coming up to me and telling me that it was much easier than what she thought.

The interesting point is that that woman, like all others during the combat application practice, was not bothered about the various steps she must do to relax and to throw a hefty man to the ground. She just relaxed and threw him, which she did elegantly.

But how did she do it? It is like asking how did she walk. She just walked. In the same way she just relaxed and threw him to the ground.

Such skills, of course, must be learnt personally from a competent teacher, who not only must have the skills himself but also can transmit the skills to his students methodically.

If that woman merely read the instructions from books or web-pages, even if the instructions were clear and she understood them well, she could neither be relaxed nor throw a hefty man.

This is one of many reasons I have so often mentioned that arts like kungfu (including Taijiquan) and chi kung need to be learnt personally from a competent teacher.

Taijiquan vs. Taijidance

Question

I have been interested in the workings of Tai Chi for a long time. However, most people consider it only a form of therapeutic exercise.

Are there any forms of Tai Chi with a focus on self-defense?

Zach, United States (September 1998)

Answer

Tai Chi Chuan, or Taijiquan in Romanized Chinese spelling, is an exceedingly effective martial art.

You will find a lot of information on Tai Chi Chuan as a martial art in my book, "The Complete Book of Tai Chi Chuan" or in my web-site.

For various reasons, Tai Chi Chuan has been so debased today that an overwhelming majority of those practicing it do not even know that it is a martial art. Interestingly, most of them call it "Tai Chi" instead of "Tai Chi Chuan" which is the proper term.

"Tai Chi" literally meaning "Grand Ultimate", is a Chinese classical term for the cosmos, and it is also used in many other disciplines such as Taoism, feng shui (or the classical study of environmental energy flow), astrology as well as other styles of kungfu.

The term "Tai Chi" in Tai Chi Praying Mantis Kungfu, for example, has nothing to do with Tai Chi Chuan.

Practicing Tai Chi Chuan is not just a therapeutic exercise, it is an excellent way to promote good health. In other words, you do not have to be sick or want to fight, in order to enjoy the benefits of Tai Chi Chuan. And good health here is not just physical, but also emotional, mental as well as spiritual (but not religious).

Nevertheless, to gain these benefits you have to practice Tai Chi Chuan, not just Tai Chi forms or Tai Chi dance.

As if to rub salt to injury, many people do not even practice Tai Chi dance; they "play" it. The expression "playing Tai Chi" is not only used in the West, but also among many Chinese in the East.

The crucial difference is that when you practice Tai Chi you go over and over again the dance like movements you have learnt so as to become a good Tai Chi dancer, whereas when you play Tai Chi you nonchalantly perform dance like Tai Chi movements to while away your time.

On the other hand, when you practice Tai Chi Chuan, you train hard, and sometimes enduringly, martial Tai Chi Chuan movements, paying attention to energy and mind, to gain good health, combat efficiency and spiritual joy.

This does not necessarily mean that playing Tai Chi is not beneficial. Indeed, for some people, like the elderly who have a lot of time to spare or businessmen and professionals who have a lot of stress, playing Tai Chi is probably more beneficial than training Tai Chi Chuan.

Genuine Tai Chi Chuan training is certainly not easy, and for most people is no fun, but for the very few who have the rare opportunity to learn from real Tai Chi Chuan masters and who are ready to invest time and effort (not merely pay lip service that they will sacrifice everything to acquire a great art) the benefits are so wonderful that they may not have thought them possible.

All forms of Tai Chi Chuan, without a single exception, focus on self-defense, otherwise it cannot be Tai Chi Chuan. The term "Chuan" in Tai Chi Chuan means martial art.

All movements in Tai Chi Chuan, including innocent-looking ones like lifting the arms up and bringing the hands back at the start and at the end of a Tai Chi Chuan set, are there for combat, and not for spectator-pleasing or even therapeutic, considerations.

Actually, while many people all over the world play or dance Tai Chi, very, very few practice Tai Chi Chuan.

Question

I have learnt various sets of movements all in the Yang style Tai Chi Chuan.

Are there any simple tests to see if what I am learning is Tai Chi Chuan or Tai Chi dance? What is the difference?
Zachary, Australia (August 1999)

Answer

Yes, here is a simple two-fold test.

One, ask yourself whether you have developed any internal force from your Tai Chi training. If you are not sure, then you have not developed any internal force. If you have — just as if you have taken your dinner, or taken a walk — you will know.

Two, spar with some martial artists of any styles. Can you put up some defenses, even if you loose in the sparring? If you do not even know what to do when someone throws a punch or a kick at you, then what your have been learning is Tai Chi dance.

If you can answer "yes" to these two questions (not just one), you are practicing Tai Chi Chuan.

Tai Chi Chuan is an internal martial art. Practicing Tai Chi Chuan gives you good health and combat efficiency.

There is nothing internal or martial about Tai Chi dance. Practicing Tai Chi dance gives you gracefulness and balance.

The two-fold test above tells you whether your training has been internal and martial.

Question

I have for the last 5 years practiced kungfu, Tai Chi and a couple of other martial arts and I have noticed something.

With the Tai Chi I have seen quite a few people (1-2 dozen) who can perform all the movements in Tai Chi with little or no difficulties (I know from experience that these movements are taxing on the legs and the mind) and have been told that Tai Chi has many benefits, one of which is physical fitness.

Yet I have seen many people with weight problems who have been practicing for years.

I have also seen people who can perform the Tai Chi movements with great ease yet cannot do a single sit up without struggling and cannot even run a few feet without wheezing.

Now I am not knocking Tai Chi as a beneficial exercise, but I do have to ask if the benefits aerobically are all that great?

Sure these people probably were not getting a fat free diet but not all the ones I have seen were overweight, just unfit.

Simon, Australia (November 1998)

Answer

Your observation is very apt. What these people practice is not real Tai Chi Chuan (spelt as Taijiquan in romanized Chinese) but a debased form, which for the sake of contrasting with real Tai Chi Chuan, I would call Tai Chi dance.

Tai Chi Chuan is an internal martial art. Hence, by definition, if someone does not have internal force and does not know combat application, he or she cannot be practicing Tai Chi Chuan.

Tai Chi dance is the external Tai Chi Chuan movements without any internal force and combat application.

The unfortunate thing is that most Tai Chi dancers do not realize they are only dancing Tai Chi external movements; many of them are in the delusion they are practicing one of the greatest martial arts of the world.

Actually today very few people practice genuine Tai Chi Chuan; most people, including those in China, do Tai Chi dancing. Some even add music to the dance.

There are many reasons why Tai Chi Chuan has degenerated into Tai Chi dance.

One reason is that there are very few genuine Tai Chi Chuan masters today.

Secondly, students are not willing to undergo the tough training that genuine Tai Chi Chuan demands. Thirdly, Tai Chi dancing schools are quite plentiful everywhere.

It is quite easy to become a Tai Chi dance student or even a Tai Chi dance instructor. If you know some external Tai Chi movements, even if you have just learnt them for three weeks, and especially if you are Chinese, you can easily start your own Tai Chi class.

In my opinion, the benefits of doing Tai Chi dance is mainly social; its health and fitness benefits are minimal.

Unlike other forms of dancing, like modern disco or classical dance drama, Tai Chi dancing does not need much stretching and vigorous actions. It is no surprise that many Tai Chi dancers cannot do sit ups or run a few feet.

But genuine Tai Chi Chuan practitioners are different.

They are not only physically fit, emotionally stable and mentally fresh, they may even become stronger and healthier as they grow older. And they do not have to go on diet, do sit ups or run a few miles to be fit. They are fit because they do chi kung, which literally means "energy work".

I have written an article on my web-site titled **Taijiquan is Not a Dance** which will provide you with some useful information on how one may convert Tai Chi dance to Tai Chi Chuan.

I wish to clarify that my answer here is not meant to belittle those who do Tai Chi dance; it is actually a sincere attempt to make them realize that in terms of health benefits and combat efficiency, they are wasting their time.

But not all is lost. If they can put some internal force and combat application into their dancing movements, they may change their Tai Chi dance into Tai Chi Chuan.

Question

Why do many students shy away from learning the fighting aspects of the art?

I for one would feel cheated if an instructor said he would not teach push hands, tai chi self defense, or san da.

Shang Wu, USA (November 1998)

Answer

One main reason is that many people, especially in the West, do not know that Tai Chi Chuan is a martial art.

Another reason is that they expected some gentle exercise for relaxation, and are not prepared for the hard work that practicing the fighting aspects of Tai Chi Chuan would demand.

Thirdly, there are few Tai Chi Chuan masters, although there may be many Tai Chi dance instructors who have given the false impression that Tai Chi is play.

Qiqong

History

Question
Could you please tell me how old chi kung is?
Robin, USA (September 2000)

Answer
The earliest piece of archaeological evidence on chi kung in extant is a piece of jade pedant with chi kung instructions craved on it describing how to attain the small universal chi flow. It is dated by archaeologists to 380 BCE.

The small universal chi flow is an advanced art where chi is circulated round the body through the ren and the du meridians. Hence more elementary types of chi kung could have existed much earlier before this date.

Chi kung historians believed that chi kung could have existed continuously till now for more than 5000 years.

Question
Where did it originate from, i.e. the country?
Robin, USA (September 2000)

Answer
Chi kung originated from China and has a continuous history till today.

"Chi kung", or "qigong" in Romanized Chinese, is actually an umbrella term referring to various arts of energy serving various purposes, such as for health, martial art, mind expansion, and spiritual cultivation.

Besides in China, various arts of energy known by different names have existed in all great civilizations of the world.

Different Types of Qiqong

Question
There are so many types out there that it gets real confusing to know which ones are the best and most powerful — especially since some give 'opposite' results.

For example, Tai Chi practice creates a body that is hard inside soft outside and Hsing-I practice creates body that is hard on the outside soft on the inside.

Jeff, USA (December 1998)

Answer

They are confusing only to those who are ignorant of their philosophy and practice. To those who know, they are crystal clear.

What is the best and most powerful for one who has properly practiced, not merely read about, qigong for many years is certainly not the best and most powerful for another who just performs gymnastics or dance.

The different types of qigong, as well as kungfu, developed because they serve different needs and abilities.

In your present situation, what serves your needs and abilities best is not the most powerful, but the simple, direct and effective, such as "Lifting the Sky" or "Carrying the Moon" as described in my books on qiqong.

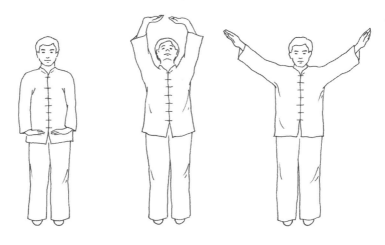

Lifting The Sky

Question

I have also heard of Chi-Lel QiGong by Master Pang Ming MD in China and Yan Xin QiGong by Dr Yan Xin MD and of course the Shaolin Chi Kung in your book.

Are they all simple, powerful, effective and enjoyable to practice?

Jo, USA (July 1998)

Answer

Grandmaster Pang He Ming and Grandmaster Yan Xin are amongst the greatest chi kung teachers in the world today. Their teachings, which range from beginners' levels to very advanced levels, not only have benefited many people but also have added much depth and dimension to chi kung.

Yes, Zhi Neng Chi Kung, Yan Xin Chi Kung and Shaolin Cosmos Chi Kung are simple, powerful, effective and enjoyable to practice.

Interestingly, and if I am not mistaken, the source of both Zhi Neng Chi Kung and Yan Xin Chi Kung is Shaolin Cosmos Chi Kung — not the Shaolin Cosmos Chi Kung that I practice but the one practiced by masters long ago.

It is worthwhile to note that "simple" does not mean simplistic.

These chi kung types are simple in the sense that they do not have unnecessary frills or padding, and as such their physical movements are easy to perform, but their effects are profound because every physical movement is a means to train energy and mind.

Question

Is advanced qin-na (the healing aspect of it) a part of qigong?
Ron, USA (May 1998)

Answer

Yes, qigong plays a very important part in qin-na, especially in its combat application.

Without internal force, which is usually developed through qigong, it is difficult to implement the "na" technique properly, such as in gripping an opponent's vital points.

Qigong also plays an important part in healing injuries caused by qin-na.

When we have caused an energy blockage in the tissues, joints or vital points of an opponent, we can remedy the injuries much faster if we employ qigong therapy.

Nevertheless, traumatology or die-da (pronounced as t'iet t'a, or tit ta in Cantonese) is probably more important in qin-na and other aspects of kungfu healing, so much so that traumatology can be called kungfu medicine. In the past, every kungfu master was also a die-da expert.

Die-da, or tit-ta in Cantonese, literally means "fall-hit"; it refers to that specialized branch of Chinese medicine that treats injury (rather than illness), especially injury due to falling or being hit.

Tit-ta is often mispronounced as thiet ta or being hit by iron.

Question

Can you please tell me something about Guolin Qigong?

Lim, Malaysia (January 2000)

Answer

Guolin Qigong was invented by the female master Guo Lin.

It resembles a form of elegant walking, and is meant to contain or overcome cancer.

It is very popular amongst cancer patients who also have found practicing qigong together regularly and sharing experiences a definite contributing factor towards their recovery.

Question

Can you please tell me something about Chan Mi Gong?

Lim, Malaysia (January 2000)

Answer

Chan Mi Gong is a school of advanced qigong incorporating the principles and practices of Chan or Zen, and Mi or Vajrayana.

Both Chan and Vajrayana are two major schools of Mahayana Buddhism, the former is popular in China and the latter in Tibet.

Although it has a rich Buddhist background, Chan Mi Gong is non-religious. Mind plays a crucial role in this school of qigong, and at the highest level it aims to help the practitioner attain spiritual enlightenment.

At a lower level, which is still more advanced than most other forms of qigong that pay attention to bodily forms, Chan Mi Gong is very effective for health and vitality.

One of its fundamental exercises is called Traveling Dragon, whereby a practitioner standing at the upright, relaxed position sends his qi up and down his spine.

Subsequently he lets this qi flow from his spine spread spontaneously to other parts of his body, or directs it to his vital organs or systems. If you can perform just this exercise well, you need not look elsewhere for the needs of your health and vitality.

As in all advanced qigong, you must learn it from a master.

If you learn from a bogus instructor or from a book or video, you will only perform its outward forms, in which case you will probably get more benefits for your health and vitality by practicing ballet or ballroom dancing.

Question

A teacher of this art claims in his web-page that his internal energy exercise called Nui Kung is much higher than chi kung.

What is Nui Kung, sifu? Is it really higher than chi kung?

Stanley, Indonesia (June 2000)

Answer

The numerous arts of kungfu force training are arbitrarily generalized into two groups, namely Nui Kung and Ngoi Kung, or internal arts and external arts.

Nui Kung (or to be more exact in its pronunciation, Noi Kung) and Ngoi Kung are in Cantonese pronunciation. In Mandarin pronunciation and Romanized spelling, they are "nei gong" and "wei gong" respectively.

One should remember that unlike scientific terms in western culture, Chinese terms are meant for convenience and therefore not exclusive.

What exactly is Nui Kung is open to various interpretations, but the common consensus is that Nui Kung involves the training of jing, shen and qi, or the internal dimensions of essence, spirit and energy.

Hence, arts like zhan zhuang (stance training), meditation and abdominal breathing would be Nui Kung. In contrast, training that involves jin, gu and bi or muscles, bones and flesh, like stretching, striking poles and hitting sandbags would be Ngoi Kung.

The term chi kung (qigong) is popularly used only recently. In the past, what is called chi kung today was called Nui Kung.

That teacher's claim can be true or false.

This is due to the limitation of words, and to the linguistic difference between Chinese and English.

What he probably meant was that he uses the term "Nui Kung" to refer to his particular energy exercise, and not as a general term referring to the whole genre of energy exercises, and that by chi kung he means some forms of external dance-like exercises, which are actually practiced by the majority of people who say they do chi kung. In this sense he is right.

But if we take the terms Nui Kung and chi kung in their actual meanings, as I have explained above, Nui Kung is chi kung.

Yet, if we wish to split hairs, Hui Kung is of a higher morphological level, but not necessarily more powerful than chi kung, because Nui Kung includes all the arts that train essence, spirit and energy, whereas chi kung refers to arts that only train energy.

Question

He also claims that to be a master of Nui Kung and you only need 3 - 6 month to learn from him and will be able to knock out 4 bigger persons in one move.

Stanley, Indonesia (June 2000)

Answer

Technically speaking, his claim can be true, but is certainly very misleading.

If you train hard almost any martial art technique specifically for 3 to 6 months, such as continuously punching a sandbag or kicking your shins against a pole, you can develop sufficient power to knock out four bigger persons in one continuous move provided your opponents are not skillful or powerful.

This, in fact, is normal in Muai Thai training. A Muai Thai fighter can knock out four or more bigger but untrained persons in one continuous move, especially when the untrained persons are so taken by the attack that they froze in their positions.

But, in my opinion, becoming such a "master" is not desirable. It would be more effective if you use an iron bar against the bigger persons.

Question

My question deals with great Grandmasters Cheng Man Ching and Yang Lu Chan. Several books described that their chi kung skills are very high and profound.

Could you please explain in details what kind of chi kung they practice?

Bodhi, Thailand (February 1999)

Answer

The Taijiquan Grandmasters Yang Lu Chan and Cheng Man Ching, naturally, practiced Taiji Chi Kung.

They did not have to practice special chi kung exercises outside their Taijiquan sets; because Taijiquan itself, when properly practiced, is a complete system of chi kung.

Every Taijiquan movement is actually a training of energy and mind. Understanding this, you will appreciate why I have frequently said that most Taiji players today perform Taiji dance and not Taijiquan.

Yang Lu Chan's favorite Taijiquan pattern is "Grasping Sparrow's Tail". Often he would practice only this pattern, and nothing else. And he would practice it continuously for hours, going over and over the same pattern thousands of times.

During his travels all over China after graduating from his master Chen Chang Xin, Yang Lu Chan used only this pattern to defeat many kungfu masters of various styles, earning the enviable nickname of Yang the Ever Victorious.

Understandably, many people, especially those who pay attention to external forms, may doubt whether it was true that Yang Lu Chan could use only one technique to defeat many masters using a great variety of techniques.

I validated this point on two separate occasions, once in Germany and another time in Spain. Although my skills and force without doubt is much, much inferior to that of Yang Lu Chan, I was able to successfully defend myself using only "Grasping Sparrow's Tail" against numerous modes of attack from an international jujitsu sparring champion.

I repeated the feat against a karate instructor in Spain.

In Portugal while commenting on the profundity in simplicity of chi kung, I cited the Chen Style Taijiquan pattern "Lazily Rolling Up Sleeves" as an example.

This was the pattern from which "Grasping Sparrow's Tail" of Yang Style Taijiquan developed.

I mentioned that if one had developed sufficient internal force from practicing this pattern, he could use only this pattern to counter virtually any attack.

This of course was hard to be believed, and accordingly many people asked if I could demonstrate.

When I consented, they unanimously chose a tough-looking but very pleasant man, whom I later learnt was a 4th dan karate master, to be my opponent.

The master attacked me in many ways, but I could effectively defend myself using only "Lazily Rolling Up Sleeves".

Actually it was not the technique in the "Grasping Sparrow's Tail"or the "Lazily Rolling Up Sleeves" pattern that was responsible for my effective defense, but the internal force developed from continuously practicing this pattern that was crucial.

In other words, if I or anyone for that matter, merely practice "Grasping Sparrow's Tail"or "Lazily Rolling up Sleeves" as a physical exercise, and without its chi kung aspect, I would be unable to use it to defend myself from a simple kick or hold even if I have practiced it for years.

Question

You mention a style called "Dragon Strength Qiqong".

Presumably this is a "hard" external style - it sounds like a nice complement to the Wahnam "soft" waidan exercises in your books and the Yi Jin Ching and Chen style Tai Chi that my own master is teaching me.

Patrick, USA (November 1997)

Answer

The "Dragon Strength" that I practice, and my Shaolin Wahnam Qiqong are both hard and soft.

The type of qigong we practice in Shaolin Wahnam School of Kungfu and Chi Kung is called Shaolin Cosmos Qigong. It is not waitan qigong.

An invaluable piece of advice I learnt from my master, Sifu Ho Fatt Nam, is that any good kungfu or qigong type should have both hard and soft, internal and external aspects.

If it is only hard or soft, internal or external, it is not an advanced art.

Shaolin Kungfu is often mistaken to be hard only, where as Taijiquan is only soft. Indeed Shaolin Kungfu, such as the Cotton Palm, can be very soft; and Taijiquan, such as the elbow strike in Chen style, can be hard.

My Dragon Strength Qiqong was developed from the "Shaolin Dragon Strength Circulating Qi" kungfu set.

At its advanced level, an exponent uses his mind to direct energy flow, and the energy flow in turn moves the body.

In other words, when the exponent wishes to execute a palm strike, for example, he merely thinks of the palm strike and it will be executed swiftly and forcefully, without using muscles.

His internal force is so fluid and powerful that it can be executed by any part of his body.

Training

Teaching from the Heart and Inspiring by Example
Leslie James Reed
Director of International Taijiquan and Shaolin Wushu Association

My name is Leslie James Reed.

I am a director of the International Taijiquan & Shaolin Wushu Association; an organization committed to offering traditional and authentic Chinese martial and health arts within our various communities around the world.

Our association is represented in Britain, Scotland, Ireland, the United States of America, South Africa, Spain, Hungary and Hong Kong.

In South Africa I represent a total of 17 schools throughout the country.

I first heard of Wong Sifu from a student who described the various books he had read by Wong Sifu in such glowing terms that I felt I had to investigate further.

I visited Wong Sifu's web-site and therein found the writings of a man who expressed so completely what I had always believed to be the true spirit and philosophy of Chinese martial and health arts.

I immediately contacted Wong Sifu and asked to be accepted on an Intensive Qigong course — I will be forever grateful that he consented to teach me.

When I arrived in Malaysia in April this year Wong Sifu was there to meet me at the airport — that act of kindness and goodwill set the tone for the rest of my stay in Malaysia.

I can honestly say that my study periods were times of extreme personal growth.

Wong Sifu is a true master (a rarity in the martial arts community of today) — he has an excellent command of the English language and offers clear and logical reasoning behind the philosophies which form the foundations of Qigong.

But Wong Sifu teaches from the heart — he inspires by example — he is the living expression of the power of Qigong.

Wong Sifu's words help to maintain the structure of my daily Qigong sessions now that I am back home in South Africa — but it is the experience of the power of his Qi which inspires me daily to keep on training.

What Wong Sifu expresses, I want — and there is no finer teacher than example.

It is thanks to Wong Sifu's comprehensive and practical teaching skills that I will one day achieve the experience and expression of Qi which is so apparent in every gesture of this true master.

I was honored to meet some of Wong Sifu's senior students in Malaysia and here again, I was able to witness Qi being manifested in a practical and clear way.

Wong Sifu also helped me to improve my Taijiquan and Kungfu training — I hope to continue this process with him in the future.

I have already received a wonderful gift — thanks to my training time spent with Wong Sifu. For over three decades I have suffered from sleep apnoea, a form of sleep disturbance which caused me great anxiety before retiring each night.

This has completely disappeared (since after my first lesson with Wong Sifu in fact) and I now wake up refreshed and energized each morning.

In October this year I and a group of my students will be visiting Wong Sifu in Malaysia for a group Qigong course — I hope to make this an annual event as I believe that Qigong is worthy of promotion as a health and lifestyle process beyond compare and that Wong Sifu is one of very few people in this world worthy of the title 'Qigong Master'.

Sifu, I want to take this opportunity of publicly thanking you for giving me the truly wonderful gift of true Qigong.

With gratitude and great respect.
Leslie James Reed
22 May 1999
E-mail: itswasa@mweb.co.za

Question

It seems hard to imagine that when we are aware of the years the monks spend in training, what we could possibly learn in a few days of your intensive chi kung course?
Jack and Steve, USA (March 1998)

Answer

You will learn in a few days what many others may not achieve in 20 years! It is hard to believe it. Let me give you just one or two examples.

Try asking politely some masters and advanced students whether they can tap energy from the cosmos and direct it to wherever they will in their body, such as to their hands, feet and stomach.

Probably they will tell you that this was a secret art of great masters, and is probably lost now although it is mentioned in books.

Ask them whether they could generate their own internal energy flow, or develop internal force.

Anybody who has access to classical texts of internal arts would have known these are fundamental skills, but unfortunately not many people have these skills nowadays.

You are going to learn these skills in my intensive course. You can learn and experience the skills in a few days, but you have to practice conscientiously for at least a few months, if not years, before these skills become lasting.

Question

I just finished reading the answers for the December(1) serial, and I am quite alarmed by your response to Jeff from USA, concerning his practice of Zhan Zhuang.

I was not aware of the possibilities of internal damage caused by its practice.

I have been practicing the Golden Bridge for the past two months, and I would like to know what are the warnings I will receive if I have been practicing incorrectly.

Max, Malaysia (February1999)

Answer

A tell-tale symptom would be pain in the chest.

If this persists, stop the exercise.

On the other hand, pain in the arms and legs are part of the developmental process.

Question

I am not under the supervision of any genuine qigong master, so I try to be careful in my practice.

I have been practicing for about 4 months now, starting with Pushing Mountains (20 times) and Lifting the Sky (10 times).

At the moment, I am practicing Lifting the Sky (20 times), Pushing Mountains (50 times) and Golden Bridge every night. It has only been two months or so since I began practicing Golden Bridge.

If you do not mind, I would like your comments or opinion on my practice habits.

Max, Malaysia (February 1999)

Answer

So long as you progress slowly, your schedule is fairly safe.

Question

Is it okay if I do not practice self-induced chi movement? I do not really enjoy it.

I do feel myself swaying but it cannot compare to the feeling of "aliveness" I get when I practice the dynamic patterns.

Max, Malaysia (February 1999)

Answer

You can do without the self-induced chi movement, but it is advisable to do it, especially at the initial stage, as a precaution against faulty practice.

Generally, self-induced chi movement is enjoyable; if you did not enjoy it, you might not have performed it correctly.

Dynamic patterns usually generate more "static" energy; this is probably the reason why you feel more "alive".

Question

Another question pertain to Golden Bridge or the Horse-riding stance.

How long or how much practice does it take to achieve 10 minutes in the stance?

After two months, I can stand just about two minutes without too much discomfort. I do not know whether to continue at two minutes until I feel no discomfort at all or to push myself constantly for more.

Max, Malaysia (February 1999)

Answer

It depends on a few variables, such as how properly and regularly you practice.

Generally, if you practice daily, you should be able achieve 10 minutes in Golden Bridge or the Horse-Riding Stance between 6 months to a year.

Two minutes of performing the Horse-Riding Stance or the Golden Bridge after two months of training is good progress.

But make sure your stance is sufficiently low.

For further progress, gently push yourself. Go for 2.1 minutes after three days, then 2.2 minute after 5 days, etc.

Do not stand up until your set time is up. A stop-watch or an alarm clock would be helpful to keep time.

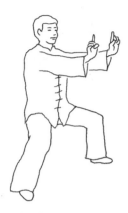

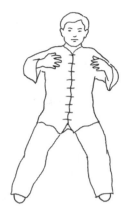

The Golden Bridge   The Three-Circle Stance

Question

I also have a slight problem which I hope you can help me with.

Last November, during a training session, my sparring partner swiped my left leg, behind and left of the knee. I did not think much about it then, but it was earlier this year, when I wanted to practice taijiquan, that it began to give me problems. I could not stand in the goat-riding stance at all; it really hurt and my leg was in constant pain.

The pain stopped me from practicing the Three Circle stance. But when I started the Horse-riding stance two months ago, it was fine, so I assumed it was healed.

It was only a few days ago, when I tried to sit in the goat-riding stance again, that I realized the pain was still there.

The pain is rather strange; it never hurts when I am walking, jumping, running, or in the Bow-Arrow stance or any of the other stances, except for the goat-riding stance.

I hope you can suggest something to help.

Max, Malaysia (February 1999)

Answer

There is some energy blockage at the spot where you felt the pain.

The position of the goat-riding stance pressurizes on the spot, aggravating the blockage. The problem can be easily overcome with self-induced chi movement.

First perform deep knee bending while on your toes about 20 times. Then go to self-induced chi movement.

While you are in the midst of the chi movement, gently think of your injured spot. Chi will flow there to help clear the blockage. Continue the chi-movement for about 15 minutes. Perform once in the morning and once in the evening or at night.

Your problem should be overcome in 2 to 4 weeks.

Question

I am wondering about another thing, Sifu.

You have often mentioned that a good book is not a substitute for a good teacher, and I have read that in a few other places too.

However, there are quite a few stories about people finding ancient qigong texts and learning from them. And even more movies, I am sure, about people fighting to get a kungfu manual or something like that.

Please do not take offense; it is not that I do not trust your word, but I would like to know whether there is any truth in those stories, fanciful as they are.

Max, Malaysia (February 1999)

Answer

Yes, the stories are true, although many of them may have been exaggerated in movies.

Sifu Zhang Zihi Tong from Taiwan, for example, found an ancient chi kung text, practiced it diligently and invented Waitankung, a school of chi kung that is very popular today, especially in South East Asia.

But these people who benefited from chi kung texts were already familiar with chi kung; the texts provided knowledge or techniques to enhance what they practiced.

Moreover, had they learnt from the masters of the texts instead, their achievement would be much more.

The big problem facing those unfamiliar with chi kung but who learn from books, is that they tend to pay attention to chi kung external forms, and miss the inner essence of chi kung.

In other words, they perform gymnastics or dance, and not energy management.

Question

Last of all, I would like to thank you, not just for taking the time to read this e-mail, but also for all the joy you brought into my life. I cannot afford your classes, so I really appreciate the fact that you decided to share your knowledge in the form of books.

Qigong has made me feel alive, vibrant and happy. Before, I was constantly depressed, easily tired and once even contemplating suicide.

Although I know qigong will never be the same without personal guidance, it does not matter. I am happy with what I have now. Life is worth living again.

Thank you, and thank you again. May your life be a long and blessed one.

Max, Malaysia (February 1999)

Answer

I am very happy that my book has helped to restore your health and bring joy to your life.

Keep up with your practice and you will gradually find that every word I have written in my book is true — words like those extolling that apparently simple chi kung exercises can bring profound benefits.

Should you have any questions, please do not hesitate to contact me, although, as in this case, it may take me some time to reply. But if your questions are urgent, call me by phone. As you gain vitality and mental freshness from your chi kung practice, you will certainly find life a joy to live.

Thank you for your sincerity.

While a good chi kung book is a poor substitute for a genuine chi kung teacher, it is certainly better than hundreds of bogus instructors who teach chi kung gymnastics or dance. While my fees are very high, some of my best chi kung is taught to deserving students without any charges.

Perhaps in future when the time is ripe you may learn chi kung from me without having to pay fees.

Question

I am a new chi kung student. I am on my own but I started to have pains in my abdomen (left side), they were sharp in nature. I went to my Doctor who said he could find nothing wrong.

Could this be caused by an "energy blockage" and how would it be possible to release this?

I also have started to lift weights in a gym. Would it be wrong to use "chi kung" methods of sending energy from the "Dan Tian" to the arms to lift the weights?

I notice that my glasses fog up when I do this.

Bill, USA (April 1998)

Answer

I am answering your question immediately instead of the normal procedure of placing your question in line (which would probably take a month or two longer to be answered), because the situation you are in seems to be urgent.

Your case is likely to be a case of energy blockage.

Your doctors would find nothing wrong because "energy" is still not in the vocabulary of conventional medicine.

Do not continue with whatever chi kung you are doing, and stop lifting weights or working out in a gym for the time being.

Instead, do the following, once in the morning and another time in the evening or at night. Practice for about ten minutes — not more. Preferably practice outdoors; if you practice indoors, do so with good air circulation.

Stand upright and be relaxed. Smile from your heart. Then perform "Lifting the Sky" about 20 times.

Refer to my book "The Art of Chi Kung" or "Chi Kung for Health and Vitality" for how to perform this exercise. (If you do not have a copy, buy or borrow one, but do not steal.)

Breathe in gently. Breathe out with some force, but do not over exert your self. If you are not quite sure what "with some force" is, it is sufficient if your breathing out is more than your breathing in.

After "Lifting the Sky" about 20 times, gently close your eyes (if they are not already close). Gently visualize or think of your energy blockage being cleared, and visualize or think of energy flowing down your legs.

Do not worry about how or why it works, where does the energy come from, what opens the blockage, or any other academic issues. Leave the academic intellectualization aside; it does not help you to overcome your problem.

Although your case can be serious if you allow it to persist, you need not worry unduly about it.

The remedial exercise I prescribed above should overcome your problems. But do not expect the problem to disappear in two or three days.

You have to practice for some time, probably for a few weeks. You will find that not only the problem has disappeared, but also you have more energy despite not having worked with weights or in a gym for some time. Then you may continue with your chi kung exercise or weight training if you like.

If you use chi kung methods to send energy from your dan tian to your arms while lifting weights, you can have better results with less effort, but you must know how to do it correctly. If you do it incorrectly, such as breathing in while exerting force, you may sustain internal injury.

If you realize that chi kung is an internal art that even masters need to spend many years to train, and you are not even a competent student, you would not be so unwise and unreasonable to think that you know enough to "be on your own" to apply chi kung to other arts.

Your foggy glasses is an indication that your self-taught knowledge on chi kung is insufficient to enable you to apply chi kung correctly, and if you do not heel the warning, you are on the way to another round of internal injury.

If you are contented with chi kung dance or gentle exercise, you can learn it from a book, but if you want genuine chi kung which you can safely and fruitfully apply to weight lifting and other aspects of your work and play, you have to learn it from a master.

You did not mention what type of chi kung exercise you did, or whether you learnt it from my books or other books.

Whatever it is, if a teacher or an author mentions that certain exercises are not to be attempted without supervision, you must follow the advice.

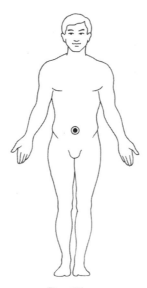

Dan Tian

Question

If you have discovered chi flow you must transport it through your whole body and the organs (I have read this) but is there an easy chi kung exercise for this, and what is that exercise?

May be you know a book or tape where this is given.

Ervin, USA (February 1999)

Answer

You do not have to transport the chi if you do not want to. Do not try this without a master's supervision; you may developed harmful effects if you perform incorrectly.

Practicing chi kung dance is easy, and sometimes you may even fool around with the dance instructor; but you have to put in a lot of hard work to practice real chi kung.

Read some of my other question-answer series.

I have given my views on learning from books and video tapes many times.

Question

What is a good exercise to let chi flow out of your PC8 point on your hand?

Ervin, USA (February 1999)

Answer

If you have the skill, any exercise can do it. If you do not have the skills, you cannot do so with any exercise at all.

An analogy is using your computer. If you have the skill, you can use computers of different brands, in different places and at different times. If you do no have any computer skills you cannot use any computer.

Question

I have been practicing the Ba Duan Jin exercises and Zhan Zhuang for the last 12 months and have experienced an improvement in my health (already good) and an increase in my energy.

As there are no high level teachers in my area I prefer to practice every day on my own and so far I have not experienced any deviations.

Alan, UK (September 1998)

Answer

Ba Duan Jin and Zhang Zhang are wonderful chi kung exercises.

By themselves, without having to learn anything else, you can attain very high levels. Not only you can have good health, vitality and longevity, you may also attain spiritual fulfillment.

If you are a martial artist, Zhan Zhuang can bring you tremendous internal force. It is simply amazing that by merely standing still at a chosen posture for some time over a long period, you can be very powerful — most people do not believe this is possible.

But if you train on your own, you must pay attention to the following points.

Practice Ba Duan Jin, or the Eight Pieces of Brocade, daily for at least six months before you attempt Zhan Zhuang, or Stance Standing.

You have to make sure you do not have any major energy blockage before starting Zhan Zhuang, and Ba Duan Jin can look after that, provided, of course, you practice correctly.

Zhan Zhuang is a powerful exercise, and is best done under supervision.

Those who practice wrongly and still persist on, may vomit blood, have deformed bodily structure, or insidiously damaged internal organs.

There are usually warning signs for wrong practice, such as discomfort, pain and nervousness.

Whenever you have such warning signs, stop your Zhan Zhuang and revert back to Ba Duan Jin. Resume Zhan Zhuang training only when the warning signs have disappeared.

If you practice Zhan Zhuang on your own, which is actually not advisable but may be attempted if you are very careful, you have to proceed very slowly; I repeat, very slowly.

If someone training with a master takes 6 months to attain certain result, you should aim at that for two years.

Question

I am studying Shiatsu and Wing Chun and would like to ask you if the type of Chi Kung I am doing is suitable for developing both healing energy for Shiatsu and Jing for martial arts?
Alan, UK (September 1998)

Answer

Yes, Ba Duan Jin is good for Shiatsu, and Zhan Zhuang for Wing Chun.

After your Shiatsu practice, flick your hands as if flicking away some water on your fingers, so as to flick out any negative energy you may have taken in from your patients.

Question

Also do I need to take any special precautions when doing the Shiatsu treatments so as to avoid giving away too much energy?
Alan, UK (September 1998)

Answer

Although some of your energy may flow into the patient, basically Shiatsu treatment involves massaging or manipulating his vital points at his soles to stimulate his own energy to flow.

This is different from treatment by a chi kung therapist who channels his energy into the patient. Hence, in Shiatsu treatment, you need not worry much about loosing your own energy.

But an urgent concern is to prevent the patient's bad energy from back-flowing to you. Thus you have to flick your hands after each practice.

Question

Usually I will do the Ba Duan Jin exercises first and then do the standing Chi Kung immediately afterwards for 20 minutes.

Is this approach correct in your view or should I modify my practice method?
Alan, UK (September 1998)

Answer

Practice only Ba Duan Jin for at least six months. Then practice Ba Duan Jin and Zhan Zhuang on alternate days, not both on the same day one after another.

After about three months, practice Zhan Zhuang every day, interspersed with Ba Duan Jin once or twice a week.

Question

Sifu for some time now I have read that Chi can be aided in speeding up the arms for strikes and I have found in a book written in the 1960s an exercise that is said to help do this.

For 15 minutes a day, every day, you sit in a relaxed position, begin breathing from the stomach with no more than 10 breaths a minute, and place your left palm over your right ear for 5 minutes, than your right palm over your left ear for another 5 minutes, and then finally combine both postures and place each palm over the opposite ear for 5 minutes, making 15 minutes total.

I was wondering if you could validate the usefulness of this exercise. Is it a truly useful exercise for developing Qi, particularly in the arms?
Cyrus, USA (January 1999)

Answer

Yes, this is a useful exercise, and you should obtain the power of chi after a few months of daily practice.

If you feel dizziness in your head, or pain in your chest as a result of this practice, stop for a few days.

You may continue when the dizziness or pain has disappeared.

Question

The author was not a Master by any means but rather a knowledgeable martial artist who collected some of the many things he had seen on his travels around the world and put them into a book.

He says its a great exercise, though I am not sure so I ask your expertise.
Cyrus, USA (January 1999)

Answer

I would say it is an effective exercise for developing powerful arms and palms, but not a great exercise for it does not give you good health, vitality, mental freshness and spiritual joy, as some chi kung exercises do, besides developing power in the arms and palms.

Question

Also, I was wondering if perhaps you would be willing to describe to me an effective exercise for developing Qi.

I am not asking for anything secretive or extremely powerful, but perhaps a basic exercise that will readily give me swifter movements, perhaps help me sleep better (definitely useful before a Calculus test!) or help me develop something better within myself that I can notice.

Something that you would have a beginner do.
Cyrus, USA (January 1999)

Answer

One of the best exercises in all chi kung is "Lifting the Sky", which you can find in my books on chi kung.

Even if you practice it at a physical level, and miss the energy and mind dimensions (which should be done under supervision), you can still attain reasonable good effects if you have the patience to practice daily for six months.

Another simple yet profound exercise is as follows.

Stand upright and relaxed, preferably in a natural, open surrounding. Breathe out gently and slowly. Then breathe in gently and slowly. It is important that your breathing should be GENTLE and slow. Repeat about 10 to 20 times.

Do this daily for six months.

Many people may not believe that such an apparently simple exercise can bring much result.

But if you can practice this daily for six months, I can safely predict that you will have swifter movements, sleep better (before and after a calculus test, and at other times) develop something better within yourself that you can notice.

Question

I am intrigued by the Cosmos Palm and would like further information on the training involved. This art seems to call to me.

I am currently learning the massage and aim to aid others to heal trauma stored in the body, facilitating the awakening to their soul as I do to my own.

Josa, USA (May 1998)

Answer

The Cosmos Palm is a wonderful art, but it is not suitable for you at present.

You must realize that a healer is one who has undergone many years of proper training under a master.

Honestly ask yourself as follows: Is this healing art capable of overcoming health problems which even people who have been professionally trained for many years like doctors and psychiatrists, cannot overcome? If so, can this healing art be acquired in a self-taught manner in a matter of a few weeks?

But more importantly you must heal yourself first. If you really want to be a healer and help others, you yourself must be healthy first, and be willing to spend a few years to undergo the necessary training.

If you are unwilling to train under a master but imagine you can become one and heal others of illness that even conventional medicine finds difficult, merely by reading some books and trying out some exercise which you yourself do not know well, you will only contribute to the rapid growth of bogus healers.

Question

Can you please tell me something about Iron Shirt Qigong?
Lim, Malaysia (January 2000)

Answer

Iron Shirt Qigong is a form of hard Shaolin Qigong, but it is also practiced in other styles of kungfu, including Tai Chi Chuan.

The main purpose is to develop a cushion of qi around the body so that the practitioner can take punches and kicks and even weapon attacks without sustaining injury, as if he were wearing an iron shirt.

The main technique is to systematically hit the body first with bean bags, then with a bundle of canes, and finally with marbles or iron granules.

It is necessary to progress gradually, otherwise one may hurt himself. It is advisable to supplement with some form of "soft" qigong, such as self- manifested chi movement, which not only overcomes internal injuries unwittingly sustained during training, but also speeds up the progress by spreading qi internally and more evenly.

If this is not available, the student should take herbal medicine once or twice a month to clear possible internal energy blockage.

While many people know the benefits of Iron Shirt Qigong, they do not realize its possible side effects, even if the art has been practiced correctly.

One major side effect is that it makes the practitioner "stiff" — not only physically but also psychically.

Considering that the ability to take bodily attacks is of little practical use whereas fluidity is very useful in our daily life, we wonder whether it is worthwhile to master this art.

Hence, while martial art instructors who stress fighting ability may consider Iron Shirt a fantastic art, most Shaolin masters do not think highly of it.

Question

What's the need for, say, Iron Palm if through chi kung a person can accomplish it?
Jack and Steve USA (March 1998)

Answer

There are different ways to achieve similar and different purposes.

If you want to break a brick with your bare hand, you may achieve this with 6 months of Iron Palm training, whereas using chi channeling may take 3 years.

If you wish to channel chi to heal others, you may achieve reasonably good result in a year with chi channeling exercises, whereas you may not be able to do so with Iron Palm even if you train for a life-time.

Question

Is it all right to practice just the second part of the "Art of Wisdom"on page 129, starting from step no 8 that is visualizing the downward and upward flow of Chi through the body and the "Oneness with Cosmos" method?

Jo, USA (September 1998)

Answer

It is all right, but you will get better result if you practice both parts — even practicing the first part for a few seconds.

Take an analogy from long jump. You may jump from the spring board, but you will get better result if you run up to the board before you jump.

Question

Can one practice Chi Kung (any kind) and Kundalini Yoga specifically Saraja Yoga at the same time?

They seem to be different routes in reaching or uniting with the Cosmos — by expanding the mind and embracing and merging with the Universe in Chi King versus awakening the coil Kundalini spiritual energy at the base of the spine in the sacrum as practiced by the Kundalini Yogi.

Jo, USA (July 1998)

Answer

I do not know much about Saraja Yoga, so I shall refer to yoga in general.

The answer to your question is yes and no, because it depends on numerous variables.

If the practitioner is familiar with both disciplines, he can practice them complimentarily. For example he could first practice chi kung dynamic patterns (like Lifting the Sky and Carrying the Moon"), then conclude with yoga meditation.

But if the objectives of his particular chi kung or yoga practice are conflicting, he should not practice them, or practice two conflicting methods in the same discipline, at the same time.

For example, practicing Submerge Breathing in chi kung, or focusing at the chakra connected with sex in yoga, enhances one's sexual performance. But this will conflict with practicing Long Breathing in chi kung to bring chi to the baihui energy field, or focusing at the crown chakra in yoga, which are useful for intellectual and spiritual cultivation.

There are many routes to reaching or uniting with the Cosmos.

Expanding the mind and awakening the kundalini are two examples, and both these routes are found in chi kung as well as yoga.

Much of raja yoga deals with expanding the mind, although yogis call the mind "spirit" and reserve the term "mind" for the intellect.

The Long Breathing in chi kung awakens the kundalini, although chi kung practitioners regard this flow of energy from the base of the spine to the top as part of a longer flow called the Small Universe.

Actually chi kung and yoga are different names for similar arts, although due to cultural, linguistic and other differences, these similar arts may have different focus and emphasis.

Question

Are there any similarities or relationships between chi kung and Hindu Chakras systems and between chi kung and the ancient Hawaii Huna systems i.e. relationships or cooperation of the Higher Self (Super-conscious Mind), Middle Self (Conscious mind) and Lower Self (Subconscious mind)?

Jo, USA (July 1998)

Answer

The chakra system in yoga is similar, but not identical, to the dan tian system in chi kung.

Both chakras and dan tians are energy fields, and are cultivated for health as well as spiritual development.

There is one noticeable difference; the major chakras are found in numerous positions along a perpendicular line from the crown of the head to the anus, whereas the major dan tians are found along the ren and du meridians round the body nearer the skin.

This difference, I believe, is because of a difference in functional emphasis.

Chi kung generally focuses more on health, whereas yoga, especially raja yoga, on spiritual cultivation.

Nevertheless, in Taoist spiritual cultivation, cultivators develop energy fields like huang ding and ni yuan which are located along the central axis like the chakra system.

On the other hand, Buddhist spiritual cultivation, especially Zen, does not pay so much attention to energy fields; it focuses directly on the mind.

I do not know much about the ancient Hawaii Huna system.

Although the terms used may be different, both chi kung and yoga deal with the subconscious, the conscious and the super-conscious mind.

Attaining "a chi kung state of mind" or "entering silence" as it was known in the past, is essential in chi kung practice if good results are to be attained.

This "chi kung state of mind" is similar to, but also surpasses, what would be called the subconscious mind.

It is a state of mind, which may manifest at different levels of depth, where the practitioner is conscious but able to use abilities which in the West would normally be referred to as belonging to the subconscious. At the deepest levels, the practitioner reaches the super-conscious or universal mind.

The division into subconscious, conscious and super-conscious mind is a western concept. Although it has some advantages, such as allowing us to understand the mind better, it is not without its setback.

For example, it may mislead many people to think (mistakenly) that these three divisions of the mind, like typical classifications in science, are exclusive, forgetting that these divisions are actually arbitrary and for the convenience of study.

Thus many people used to such categorical thinking, referred to as dualistic in Zen, find it difficult to comprehend and subsequently appreciate that it is perfectly possible to experience the subconscious or super-conscious when one is still in the conscious mind.

Question

I did a course with you and, first of all, would like to thank you for your wonderful teaching; I will never forget it.

During the course I had an experience that I told you about at that time and you just told me that I had practiced well and smiled.

What happened was that I was sitting in seiza hearing you and thought about an energy field around you. All of a sudden my body got very straight, images started to dissolve (as my ego) and the sound of the heart beat was going louder and louder. I came back afraid of where I was going.

Well, things like that happen some times in my life. Even with the arrival of the Kundalini energy coming up, I always stopped it, because both I was afraid and also thinking I was not prepared for it.

What I respectfully ask from you is if you think if I shall have these experiences in future should I trust them and go with the flow.

What I feel is that some experiences are dangerous if you stick to them, getting "THE FINGER FOR THE MOON" but on the other hand, they are probably important for your spiritual maturity. Am I right?

Joao, Portugal (April 1998)

Answer

Both your chi kung and kundalini experiences are wonderful, indicating that you have practiced well.

So long as the experiences come naturally from your practice, and so long as your practice is correct, you need not worry nor be afraid.

One sure way to tell whether you have been practicing correctly is your feeling after the practice.

If you feel well and pleasant the practice is correct; if you feel uncomfortable and unpleasant the practice is incorrect, although sometimes correct practice may produce some pain when your energy flow is attempting to break through blockages.

If you keep up your practice your experiences may occur again. When they happen, just be natural — what the Taoist say "wu-wei". Sometimes the breakthrough may be dramatic and even painful, but you need not worry about it.

Yet, you are correct about the saying "mistaking the finger for the moon". The breakthrough or the kundaline, even though the experience may be extraordinary, is actually a symptom that you are making progress; it is not the real effect for which we practice chi kung.

In other words, what we aim at are good health, vitality, mind expansion and spiritual development, and not just experiencing wonderful breakthroughs, kundalinis or other remarkable occurrences , although they do indicate that you are progressing correctly.

Question

Dear Sifu,

How are you? Some days ago, I got a phone call from Han. He was a member of the group course, the one with the autoimmunity disease.

He asked me if it was possible to do the qigong sitting.

Liong Hoo, Holland (January 1999)

Answer

It is best to do whatever chi kung or kungfu (including Taijiquan) exercises according to the way they are taught, including the way the practitioner stands, sits, lies down or moves about.

This is because the established form is the one that will give the best benefits, after the form has been evolved by masters through many centuries of development.

This does not necessarily mean one must not make any modification to the established form.

There should be at least two conditions for modification, namely the modification is necessary or will contribute to more benefits for a particular situation, and the one making the modification clearly knows what he is doing (which means he is already very familiar with the established form and is aware of some shortcomings in the form).

Question

Because of his illness, he can hardly stand more than a few minutes.

During the course he said he forced himself to stand.

The next few days he said the pain in both his legs were so severe that he could only do the qigong exercises standing for a few minutes.

Liong Hoo, Holland (January 1999)

Answer

This is an example where modification to the established form is necessary.

His pain was the result of chi accumulated from his chi kung practice, but as there are severe blockage his chi could not flow, thus resulting in pain. There is a saying in Chinese medicine as follows: "shang qi tong, shang xue zhong", i.e. "injury to chi results in pain, injury to blood results in swelling".

Blockage of energy flow is an example of injury to chi.

If this continued, it would lead to blockage of blood flow, resulting in swelling. This might lead to further complications, such as interrupting the flow of chi to and from the "heart" — which is the Chinese way of saying interrupting the flow of feedback-impulses and instruction-impulses to and from the brain or consciousness.

This may lead to the malfunction of glands and eventually organs.

Treating the swelling or treating the affected organ, as is normally the case in conventional medicine, is only treating the symptom, or at best treating a later developmental stage of the disease.

In Chinese medicine, the physician treats the root cause, which is blockage of energy flow. This can be achieved through herbalism, acupuncture, physiotherapy and massage therapy. But practicing chi kung is the most holistic and natural.

Had Han told me his problem during the course, I would have recommended some dynamic exercises to loosen his leg muscles first.

This is an example that one who starts teaching chi kung soon after he has learnt it, would be unable to make such a recommendation.

Any instructor must have practiced his art long enough to have a direct experience of its effect, as well as know enough of its background philosophy before attempting to instruct others.

Question
As I remembered a case you mentioned in one of your books, I told him he could, if it was necessary, do the qigong while sitting, but I said I would ask Sifu for sure.
Liong Hoo, Holland (January 1999)

Answer
You have done the right thing, both in telling him to do the chi kung exercise while sitting, and saying you would ask me.

A better approach is to leave dynamic patterns for the time being, but do self-manifested chi movement.

He may, if it is necessary, do the preliminary (physical) exercises of the self-manifested chi movement while sitting, but he should as far as possible enjoy his chi flow while standing so that the chi will better flow to his legs.

Question
He said the days after the course, both legs were looking very bad. There were many red spots with liquid coming out.

He showed to Paul (course member, the anesthetist}and Paul said the illness was coming out as a reaction to the qigong.

So he continued to do the qigong, and to maximize the results, he tried to do the qigong at midnight.
Liong Hoo, Holland (January 1999)

Answer
Paul is right. It is good to do qigong at midnight, but Han must not over practice. He has to give himself time for the qigong effect to take place.

Question

Han told me that because the pain was more severe, and he had to take more pills to suppress it, he felt so depressed and desperate.

I could only answer by saying, "Have faith, continue to do the qigong, the disease will be cured finally."

He already has this disease for about 10 years, so we should not expect it to be cured in an instant.

Liong Hoo, Holland (January 1999)

Answer

Instead of taking pills he can try doing self-manifested chi movement. Besides overcoming his physical problems, qigong will also overcome depression, desperation and other emotional problems.

Your advice that he should have faith and patience in his qigong practice is excellent.

Question

About myself, I am glad the intestines are not bothering me anymore. Now I am doing qigong twice a day, about 30 minutes.

I have found out that I reacted badly after eating fish and seafood, also after eating banana. So I avoid eating those things for the time being.

Later after progressing in my qigong exercises, I am sure I can eat those foods again.

Liong Hoo, Holland (January 1999)

Answer

I am glad you have progressed.

You are perfectly right. The following information will be useful for your further progress.

There are different levels of cleansing. Most people perform far below their potential. I do not know the exact percentage; the following are just hypothetical figures but the basic philosophy is the same irrespective of the figures quoted.

Let us say most people perform at 55 percent of their potential. In other words, even if 45 percent of the chi flow in your intestines is blocked, your intestines can still perform their functions and you are not clinically sick. It is worthwhile to note that in qigong, we work at the most fundamental level, i.e. the energy (or qi) level; we do not have to worry about grosser levels.

In other words we do not have to worry about the intermediate agents that cause the 45 percent blockage — we do not have to worry whether the below-par functioning is caused by a bacterial infection, an emotional attack, a structural disorder, or an excessive production of harmful chemicals from certain food. This does not mean that knowing the intermediate causes is not useful.

For example, if you know that your intestinal problem is caused by some harmful bacteria, and you have the antidote against the bacteria, taking the antidote (assuming that it does not have serious side effects) is more effective than doing qigong.

For some reasons, such as eating seafood or banana which may produce harmful chemicals inside your body, the blockage in your intestines increases from 45 to 51 percent.

Then you would have a clinical intestinal problem because your intestine functioning at 49 percent is below the 55 percent threshold level.

By practicing qigong, you cleanse away the blockage, reducing the blockage from 51 percent back to 45 percent. Hence your problem disappears, without having to take any medication. This is the first level of cleansing, and for convenience I call it the disease-elimination level.

Performing only at threshold level, i.e. 55 percent, is not comfortable. If you are not careful, such as eating some seafood or are exposed to other causes, your intestinal performance may go down below the threshold and a clinical intestinal disorder will appear again. This is not a relapse of your former disorder, but actually a surfacing of a new one.

So you continue practicing qigong and further cleanse away the blockage from, say, 45 to 35 percent. Now your intestines perform at 65 percent of their potential, 10 percent above threshold level. I call this the buffer level. You have a buffer of 10 percent.

Even if you eat seafood or are exposed to other factors which would in the past cause you intestinal disorder, now you are still free from the problem.

But if you eat seafood excessively or if the accumulated bad effects from many factors go beyond the buffer of 10 percent (i.e. for any reason, the blockage rises back from 35 to 45 percent) the intestinal disorder will again appear as a clinical disease.

If you do nothing about it and allow the blockage to increase further, say to 60 percent, you will obviously need more time and do more qigong to effect a recovery. This is the case with Han.

The explanation here is much simplified. In reality, the cause may not be direct. It can be indirect and can be multiple, such as a gland failing to produce a chemical needed by the intestines, or a lack of some trace elements needed for the production of the chemical, or an interruption of a flow of signals far way from the intestines but eventually connected to intestinal functioning. Usually it is a mixture of a few factors.

In other words, a blockage of qi flow at the intestines is not necessarily and solely caused by a physical blockage at the intestines; it can be caused by many other factors.

A Chinese physician would refer to intestinal problems as "xiao chang qi bu zu", which is "insufficient energy at the intestines".

It is not, as many Chinese unfamiliar with Chinese medical concepts might translate to their non-Chinese friends, "insufficient air at the intestines". Qi or energy in Chinese medicine is often manifested as "function".

But, as mentioned earlier, we need not worry about the intermediate causes because we work at the root cause. So long as we restore the harmonious energy flow at the intestines, the intestines will restore their natural functions.

It is significant to note the word "natural" here. We aim to restore the natural functions of the intestines, which will include digesting all types of food without trouble. We do not aim to make the intestines perform unnatural or supernatural functions, such as digesting iron nails or being able to hear sounds.

"Restoring harmonious qi flow", which means restoring natural functions, is a perfectly natural thing to do, and has been done for centuries by Chinese physicians.

There is nothing fantastic or incredible about it; it appears incredible only when people, including many Chinese, do not understand the underlying concepts and mistakenly take qi to mean air.

This also illustrates a great advantage Chinese medicine has over conventional western medicine. Western medicine often treats the symptoms instead of the cause. For example, if you complain of intestinal pain, a western doctor would give you a pain killer; if you complain of indigestion, he would give you some digestive chemicals.

If you tell him that your problem occurs after taking seafood, he would ask you not to take seafood. You and the doctor know that this may remove the symptoms but not the disease. Indeed more and more doctors are now accepting the working definition of medicine as the management of disease, and not necessarily its cure.

Chinese medicine, on the other hand, treats the patient, not just the disease. A Chinese physician is not so bothered about the symptoms of the disease or the agents that cause these symptoms. He is mainly concerned with restoring the natural functions of the patient, which in Chinese medical terminology is restoring harmonious energy flow.

This is a great advantage because whereas the western doctor works with unknown factors, attempting to find out what among the countless agents outside the patient have caused the symptoms, and if he cannot find the agent he often does not know what to do; the Chinese physician works with known factors, attempting to find out which energy systems in the patient have malfunctioned.

If, for example, he finds that the cause of the intestinal disorder is due to excessive "heat" from the colon system, he can restore the harmonious chi flow at the intestines by reducing the excessive "heat". If the cause is due to insufficient chi from the spleen system, the intestinal disorder can be overcome by increasing the spleen system chi.

Qigong is even better.

Chinese physicians working with acupuncture, herbalism, massage therapy or other Chinese medical practices have to find out the specific cause of disharmonious energy flow.

Hence, diagnosis is of utmost importance. But in qigong, diagnosis is not even needed! This is because the qi acquired in qigong practice flows holistically. Like water, energy flows from high energy areas to low energy areas, and low energy areas are health problem areas.

The area with the lowest energy level, which is the area with the most severe health problem, will receive the extra qi first, followed by the next lowest area and so on. In other words, when you practice qigong, your health problems will be overcome in the order of their seriousness.

The interesting thing is that you may not consciously know about some of these health problems, but you need not have to know, qi will work on them all the same.

Let us now return to the various levels of cleansing, which will further show the advantage of qigong over other healing systems.

Attaining the disease-elimination level of cleansing, which is the main concern of conventional western medicine and other healing systems, will overcome the disease clinically.

Attaining the buffer level, which can be achieved by some healing systems like acupuncture and massage therapy, provides a reasonable level of good health.

Qigong goes beyond this buffer level, but other healing systems do not.

Lets say you reduce the blockage further so that your intestines now can perform at 80 percent of their full potential. By this time the energy would have flowed to other systems too, because the whole energy system of the body (and mind) is closely connected.

This means all your systems can function at a high level near to the full potential. I call this the vitality level.

At the vitality level you are not only free from illness, and can eat whatever food you like to eat, you are full of vitality for daily living.

If you eat seafood or are exposed to other harmful agents, your performance may drop a few percent, but if you are normally performing at 80 percent, a drop to, say, 75 percent is marginal and you will still be considered as full of vitality by ordinary people who habitually perform at 55 percent.

Qigong practitioners who have attained the level of vitality are not sick, not because disease-causing agents do not attack them, but because these agents are eliminated long before the body function has dropped beyond the threshold level.

Beyond the vitality level is what I call the longevity level. Continued qigong practice will purify the body so that there is little blockage, and you can perform at or near full potential level, say 90 percent and above.

As soon as new blockage arises, it is cleansed away by the harmonious energy flow.

Hence all your organs are not only fit and healthy now, they will also last a long time. By nature the potential life span of a human being is around 120 years. If you have attained the longevity level of qigong, you should easily live to 80 and beyond.

It is also helpful to know the following.

When you have attained the disease-elimination level, you would have overcome your disease. But as you continue your qigong training, further cleansing in deeper levels may bring out other disease-causing factors that result in symptoms of the disease.

In other words you may think that you have a relapse of the disease as the disease-causing toxins rise to the surface from deeper levels as the result of deep cleansing.

When you have gone beyond the buffer level, all or at least most of the toxins would have been rooted out. Some toxins may still remain, but they are insufficient to cause any disease symptoms at the vitality level.

Question

A few days ago in the evening, I do not know why, but I lost my temper. This has not happened before.

My brain is still feeling confused about it. But do not worry, I am working on it with qigong.

I am very grateful to you Sifu, for giving me a weapon to overcome these problems. Thanks. The kids and Chuen are also doing well.
Liong Hoo, Holland (January 1999)

Answer

The outbreak of temper may be due to some blockage at the liver system. This can happen at the disease-elimination level or the buffer level. But I am sure you will soon overcome it, or may be have overcome it already.

I have written to Kay about the importance of practicing over learning. I am reproducing the relevant part below for you as I think you and Chuen will benefit from it.

(The following is reproduced from a personal letter to Kay and Jean of Canada.)

"My sifus, Sifu Ho Fatt Nam and Sifu Lai Chin Wah, encouraged me to learn from other teachers. That was quite logical, for Sifu Ho Fatt Nam himself had learnt from seven masters, and Sifu Lai Chin Wah had learnt from three.

But they also advised me not to spend too much time learning; instead, I should spend my time practicing.

Superficially, these two points of learning from more teachers, and of not spending too much time learning may appear contradictory.

Actually they are not; the apparent contradiction is due to the limitation of words, and also to the provisional use of language.

Words (because of their innate limitation) cannot convey fully what a speaker wants to say; and what is said (in words) is provided for that particular occasion (and may not apply to another occasion).

When I was in Spain recently I had an interesting experience which I wish to share with you.

Similar thoughts had occurred to me previously, but it was then that these thoughts came to me in a focused crystallized form. I was then sitting on a sofa watching Douglas practicing kungfu.

It suddenly dawned on me that on a few occasions I really did not know what to teach some of my close students.

It would appear odd, because I have so much to teach; I have, for example over a hundred kungfu sets and over a hundred chi kung exercises. But I knew it was not odd, and I knew the reason.

On that occasion, I recalled my time with you in Toronto, and also my time with you in Malaysia.

When I was in Toronto I wanted to teach you something new, but even though I searched hard from my very extensive repertoire I could not find anything to teach you which I knew would add to your progress.

When you were in Malaysia, I wanted to teach you something new, even as a souvenir, but I knew very well that had I done so, I would hinder your progress instead of promoting it.

In other words, there may be so many things I can teach, but I know without doubt that you will benefit more by continuing with your present practice instead of learning anything new. I told Douglas about my realization.

He told me, which I quite expected, that he was actually happy I did not teach him anything new. He said he had learnt enough techniques; what he wished to do was to practice and practice.

Although they may hold different views on many other things, almost all masters will agree that the key to becoming a master is practice. The crucial point between learning and practicing is that learning involves new things, whereas practicing involves what you already know.

My two masters did advise me on practicing in place of learning, but as I did not have the maturity of thought and depth of experience then as you and Douglas now have, I did not fully appreciate the significance of my masters' advice although I did understand its verbal meaning.

Had I followed their advice then, I would have certainly attained my present level in less than half the time."

Question

Many "mysterious" illnesses appeared - losing 30 pounds in one month, jaundice, symptoms reminiscent of epilepsy ... yet doctors could not find any cause.

Through years of erratic and violent mood swings I alienated myself from everyone... I am experimenting with visualizations or concentrations of energy inflating my body and squeezing this energy into my body.

Josa, USA (May 1998)

Answer

Chi Kung masters (real masters, not self-taught impersonators) have warned that visualization and concentrations of energy must be done with a teacher's supervision, yet you are so unwise as to experiment with these practices.

Question

I think I have a tremendous amount of chi, that is, energy that I have been building through time by concentration. My question is how can I use it properly.
Eric, Canada (December 1998)

Answer

Use it for good, and never for evil.

This may appear to be a simple and even trite statement, and you may think it does not answer your question, but I can tell you, in my capacity as a chi kung grandmaster, it is one of the best pieces of advice you can ever have.

Question

The two qigong practices I have picked to start practicing are Zhan Zhuang and Ba Duan Jin. Any comments or suggestions on these practices?
Jeff, USA (December 1998)

Answer

Zhan Zhuang, which means stance training, is a genre of powerful qigong exercises.

It is the single most widely used genre by kungfu masters of various styles, including Shaolin, Taijiquan, Bagua and Hsing Yi, to develop internal force.

But it is not suitable for beginners, especially those without the personal supervision of competent instructors.

It looks easy, as you remain in the same static position for a long time. It is easy for you to make mistakes, and easy not to realize the mistakes. Because Zhan Zhuang exercises are powerful, the adverse effects of the mistakes are potent.

Even in the unlikely situation that you do not make a single mistake in your long period of training, but if you have substantial blockage in your body to start with, the accumulated energy derived from Zhan Zhuang would cause internal injuries.

Ba Duan Jin, which is pronounced as "P'a T'uan Jin" and not as "Ba Duan Jin", and which means "Eight Pieces of Brocade", is a set of eight dynamic qigong exercises.

It is a wonderful set and is very popular today, although most people today practice it, like they practice other qigong exercises, as physical exercise rather than as qigong, which is energy exercise.

But even if they practice only the physical aspects of Ba Duan Jin, and missing its qigong dimension, there are many benefits, such as loosening muscles, promoting blood circulation and relaxation.

It does not have the adverse effects of orthodox western exercises like forcing the organs to overwork and depositing much toxic waste in the body cells. It is an ideal type of exercise for you to practice on your own.

Without the personal guidance of a qigong master, you would not obtain the wonderful qigong benefits of Ba Duan Jin, but at least you would not have serious side effects from wrong practice.

Question

I did try the 2 qigong practices you recommended in your first Qigong book for approximately 2 months (20 repetitions of each exercise), but barely felt any energy flow, increased energy, etc.

I was following the instructions to the word and was wondering why I did not feel much.

I know 2 months is not much time but I thought I would at least feel the energy enough to know that it was not my imagination. I really wanted to try to reach the induced chi flow state you mentioned — so I was disappointed when I could not get any 'results' with the preliminary practices.

Jeff, USA (December 1998)

Answer

The reason is that as you learnt from a book instead of from a master, you merely performed the physical movement of the exercises, and missed their qigong effects.

In other words, you performed qigong gymnastics or dance instead of qigong.

Virtually every one who has taken a qigong course from me, felt unmistakable qigong effects such as internal energy flow and increased energy level on the very first day. It is not for no reason that my students pay a comparatively high fee for my lessons.

Interestingly, immediately following your e-mail, is an e-mail from one of my students describing his experiences from my lessons.

He learnt from me for only a few hours — during a workshop at the Second World Qigong Congress where I was lucky to receive the "Qigong Master of the Year" award.

I am posting his questions and my answers after yours for your perusal.

Question

Two other Qigong practices I have been looking at to add to my growing list of practices, are Yi Chin Ching and Bone Marrow Washing.

Could you explain the results of these practices and comment on them? *Jeff, USA (December 1998)*

Answer

Yi Jin Jing, or Sinew Metamorphosis, is an advance qigong exercise in Shaolin Kungfu.If you practice it without proper supervision, you are likely to injure yourself.

Bone Marrow Washing is reputed to be taught by the great master Bodhidharma to the monks at the Shaolin Monastery, but there have been no records of what the techniques were both inside and outside the monastery.

From indirect evidence, I believe it could be some form of advance self-manifested qi movement whereby the practitioner channels his energy to cleanse his brain and nervous system.

In Chinese medical philosophy, the bone marrow flows into and from the brain; and corresponds in functions to the nervous system in western medical terminology.

In my recent qigong teaching trip to Austria, when we did advance induced qi flow in a class in Guttenstein, many of my students reported that they clearly felt qi cleansing their nerves and their brain.

It was certainly not imagination.

Asking them how they knew it was qi cleansing their brain is like asking someone eating an apple how he knew he was eating an apple. They knew from direct personal experience.

If you had never eaten an apple before, you might think it was not possible to eat an apple.

An expert in Yi Jin Jing, without having to undergo any hard conditioning, can have the power to kill a bull with just one strike. An expert in Bone Marrow Cleansing is very quick and accurate in his physical as well as intellectual response. Both are of course healthy, fit and full of vitality.

By "expert" I refer to someone who has trained the respective art devotedly for many years; not someone who has learnt the techniques, even if the techniques are correct, in a week-end course from an instructor who himself is incapable of such attainment.

Again, you should have due respect for such advance arts. Do not imagine you can attain similar results by merely learning from books.

Question

When practicing Zhan Zhuang to get the full benefits of this form of Qigong, do you eventually need to start mentally moving energy around your body—i.e. microcosmic, macrocosmic, etc. or will that take care of itself?
Jeff, USA (December 1998)

Answer

As Zhan Zhuang is a genre of qigong, there are many types of Zhan Zhuang exercises.

Generally the practitioner does not intentionally move qi around his body; he merely remains at his stance thinking of nothing and doing nothing.

Sometimes, for specific purposes, a practitioner may channel his qi in some specific directions, such as along his arms or down his legs.

Question

Also, will just standing eventually (without visualizing anything) allow you the ability to move chi around mentally at will without having to do any breathing or moving techniques.
Jeff, USA (December 1998)

Answer

The answer is yes and no.

In theory, everyone has the power of mind over energy and matter, which means that not only you can move your energy to flow anywhere you wish inside your body, you can also, by an act of will power, move the shoes you are wearing to the top of your friend's head.

In practice, most people have lost this natural ability. Most qigong dancers, for example, cannot even start their own energy flow, which is actually a basic skill in qigong training.

If you have the skill, you can move your qi around mentally at will without having to do any breathing techniques or moving techniques while you are in any position, at Zhan Zhuang or otherwise.

This is not a difficult skill to acquire if you are properly trained. In fact many of my students can do it after just one qigong course with me.

But they usually do it while not at a Zhan Zhuang pose, for doing so would defeat the main purpose of Zhan Zhuang, which is accumulating qi and not circulating qi.

Question

I enjoy practicing Lifting the Sky, Pushing Mountains, and Carrying the Moon the most.

I have been using these three (alternating days between dynamic and self manifested chi flow - followed by abdominal breathing and standing mediation) and feel fantastic.

Occasionally, I will change to other forms (both Shaolin Cosmos Chi Kung forms and other styles I have learnt) so I would not loose them form my memory.

John, USA (December 1998)

Answer

These three dynamic patterns are amongst the best in chi kung. That is why I have chosen them to teach my students.

Your program of alternating between dynamic patterns and self manifested chi flow, followed by abdominal breathing and standing meditation is excellent.

Generally, when one has some illnesses to be overcome, he should emphasize self-manifested chi movement.

As he progresses, he may shift his emphasis to dynamic patterns. When he is quite advance, he may spend most of his training time in abdominal breathing.

While meditation is important in every stage of chi kung training, it is crucial in the highest of chi kung achievement.

It is also advisable to occasionally practice other forms of chi kung that you have learnt so as to maintain them in your chi kung repertoire.

You will find that the fundamental skills you have acquired in your basic chi kung program will enhance your other forms of chi kung.

Question

But, I always return to these three forms because I like how I feel during and after the practice the best. I do not have any illness that I am aware of, so I use these forms to increase and maintain my energy and health.

Interestingly, I have noticed that when I am walking, I feel the chi swaying in my arms and hands — I simply smile. I have a feeling I am developing powerful hands and even more graceful martial arts movements during my martial arts practice.

More importantly, I feel a greater sense of peace and joy throughout the day.

Thank You!!!

John, USA (December 1998)

Answer

While these three forms suit you best in your present stage, later when you are more advance you could change to abdominal breathing as your main training form.

You will know when to make the change because the knowledge and experience gained in your progress will enable you to.

Your experience of chi even when you are not formally practicing chi kung is a normal chi kung development and an indication that your practice is correct. It is also an indication that you are practicing high quality chi kung.

In low quality chi kung, one needs to practice for an hour or more per session, and feels the chi kung effects only during the practice.

In high quality chi kung, one needs to practice only about 15 minutes per session, but feels the effects the whole day.

You will not only be powerful and graceful in your martial art performance, you will achieve better result in whatever you do.

This is expected because your high quality chi kung training has developed both your energy and mind.

Question

"Wang Xiang Zhai, the founder of I-Chuan, was also well known for talking in terms of force vectors and so forth in exactly the same way, saying that most people are distracted by all the talk about Qi and "nine this" and "five that" and he went right to it."

Graham, Ireland (November 1998)

Answer

I am not sure what the author wishes to say.

But I am quite sure that what Sifu Wang Xiang Zhai meant was "do not just talk about qi; do real qigong and get the practical result".

Question

I also practice 5 Animal Frolics, but I see that you have another outlook on how they should be practiced.

Am I wasting my time by doing them from the stationary posture and not from the induced Qi flow. How can other qigong masters be incorrect?
Michael, country not mentioned (December 1997)

Answer

There are two major views regarding the Five Animal Frolics.

The older view is that Hua Tuo invented this famous chi kung exercise after observing the movements and characteristics of the tiger, bear, deer, monkey and bird.

Proponents of this view generally perform the exercise as dynamic patterns or "dao yin" in Chinese.

Another view, popularized after collaborating with some recently discovered documents and archeological findings, purports that the movements, mainly self-manifested, came first, and Hua Tuo classified the great variety of movements into five main groups symbolized by the movements of the five animals.

Proponents of this view generally perform the exercise as self-manifested chi movement, or "zi fa dong gong" in Chinese.

Personally I favor the second view, and have found that practicing the exercise as self-manifested chi movement more powerful and effective in overcoming illnesses.

The choice is arbitrary; it is improper to say which approach is correct or wrong.

Question

I would like to ask if you can send me chi. I ask mainly out of the sole fact that I need it. I know from personal experience in my esoteric pursuits that the things you talk about in your book are real.

I would like to ask for your help in my healing.
Mike, Germany (December 1997)

Answer

What you need is not transmitted chi from me but acquiring chi yourself from the cosmos by practicing appropriate chi kung exercises. A good suggestion is to perform a set of self-manifested chi movement exercise described in my book for about 15 minutes every day for three months.

Then, for the next three months practice daily just "Lifting the Sky" for about 20 times, followed by Standing Meditation for about 5-10 minutes.

In six months' time you will personally experience what I mean by saying that chi kung promotes good health.

Question

I have always been interested in martial arts and chi kung.

I am currently suffering from several health problems caused by what I think is wrong chi kung practice.

Since I was disturbed during a chi kung meditation I have always been nervous and afraid, and sometimes I experience uncontrollable movements.
Azman, Malaysia (February 1998)

Answer

You are right in saying that your health problems were caused by wrong chi kung practice.

The good news is that the problems can be overcome and you can continue with proper chi kung training which will bring wonderful benefits.

Your problems were the result of what is known in chi kung terminology as "shattering of mind leading to disorderly energy flow". The shattering was caused by lost of mental control due to mental disturbance, added by fear and anxiety. Some energy is trapped within pockets of blockages. Sometimes the trapped energy flows within the confines of the blocked pockets, causing uncontrollable physical movements.

The mind has not recovered completely from its initial shock, and therefore exists in states of fear and nervousness.

The therapeutic approach is to attack the problems at their roots, and this consists of opening the blockages to release the trapped energy, as well as calming and focussing the mind.

These can be done by you yourself practicing appropriate remedial exercises, or by a master opening the blockages and calming the mind, or by the combined efforts of both.

Question

What would you suggest I do about doing Chi Kung in a noisy place. You see I live with a room mate and by a noisy street so I get distracted quite easily.
Mike, USA (July 1998)

Answer

Wake up half an hour earlier each day, go to the nearest park or garden and practice your chi kung there. The benefits you will get will far outweigh your effort or trouble.

Qiqong: A Cure for Degenerative Diseases

Overcoming Cancer and Experiencing Happiness from Within

Laura Fernandez Garrido
Air Hostess, Spain

In January 1997 my gynecologist gave me a diagnosis of breast cancer. I suffered two surgeries, and received chemotherapy and radiotherapy.

Besides, in February my partner finished our relationship.

I got two shots at the same time. My emotional crisis was for me as serious as the cancer disease.

In April I began to practice Tai Chi Chuan and chi kung. My instructor recommended me to have a personal consultation with Sifu Wong in his visit to Spain in May to look after the seriousness of radiotherapy in my lungs.

I met Sifu Wong in a park in Madrid and he explained to me what to do about my lung and my emotions "Always smiling from the heart," he said. He announced to me that in my next medical test I would be in good health, and he asked me to inform him by e-mail.

Soon I passed my medical tests and everything was all right.

I feel that my work with energy has saved by body, my mind and my soul.

My lung capacity is now much bigger than ever and I have not been sick since those years, not even influenza. My vitality is great and I am much happier now than ever, and my happiness is coming from inside and has nothing to do with external events.

Of course I practice chi-kung everyday since I met Sifu Wong.

Since 3 month ago I am teaching Shaolin Wahnam Chi Kung, following the instructor-training program of Sifu Wong. I am very happy to see my pupils too are getting a lot of benefits.

For example, after practicing for 15 days Carmen got back her menstruation that was missing one year and a half ago, even she is under 40. Besides she is getting rid of her fibromialgia pains one by one, and enjoying much more life.

Esther stopped smoking easily when she decided to do so after talking about objectives in daily life one day during a chi kung class. Now she is trying not to get angry.

Ana feels more vitality and relaxation and the energy warming her hands and body.

Pepa keeps calm even in a time of problems.

Consuelo got rid of her back pains and sleeps well since she began the practice. She received a tax inspection and began to do chi kung instead of to panic. She remained calm as she could not imagine before.

Angeles felt more strength in her body and in her mind. She is recovering self-esteem an expressing her opinions with more self-confidence.

Thanks, Sifu.

Laura
Madrid
18 April 2000

Excellent Exercise to Overcome Cancer

Pilar Fernandez

Pilar Fernandez
Girona
Espaha

Mr. Wong Kiew Kit
Shaolin Wahnam Chi Kung Institute
Sungai Petani, Kedah
Malaysia
July 13th 1999

Respected Teacher Wong,

Thank you very much for the treatment that I received from you three years ago. The exercises that you taught me in 1996 were excellent for me.

I do not know if you remember me. My name is Pilar Fernandez. I live in Girona, Spain.

I had the opportunity of meeting you in Castellon, Spain in September 1996.

At that time I had been operated from utero and ovaries cancer and I had metastasis in three limphatic ganglions. You were kind enough to check-up on me in your spare-time during a short kungfu course that you were doing there.

You met my sister-in-law's brother in Sevilia in February 1999. His name was J. A. (full name omitted for ethical reason). He had cancer too. He told me, after he saw you, that you like to receive news from people that you have treated. Hence, I am writing you now. Unfortunately J. A. died in May.

The appointment with you was very important for me. You gave me hopes to overcome my illness.

For many months, the only moment during the day that I felt sure that I would not die was when I did my qiqong exercises. Moreover in a few times all my medical tests have returned to normal. I have been feeling better every day during all this time. Now I do Chi-Kung one time a day. I like to do it.

I hope to have the opportunity of seeing you again in your next visit to Barcelona.

I always will be very grateful to you. Our planet is a better place thanks to teachers like you.

Thank you very much.

Pilar Fernandez

Question

I am one of your students in the your qigong course.

Daily I practice qigong in the early morning, 6:15 am to 6:50 am in a housing estate park.

Every 3 months I go to a hospital for a routine cancer checkup. In the last checkup the result shows that I have cancer reoccurrence after 15 months of free cancer.

The doctor advises surgery and then chemo treatments (about 3-6) using a very powerful drug, Taxol.

Here is the brief story.

In April 1998 I was diagnosed with ovarian cancer. Subsequently I went for surgery (hystermony - removing the ovaries, tubes and the womb).

After about one and half month of rest, I started chemo treatment using standard drugs for 8 courses and in early December I was given a clean bill of health; until now.

Sifu, please advise .

Now the cancer tumour is in the vagina; blood test is normal.

If I go for surgery, when can I practice qigong and what are the forms to use and for how long. Then also during the chemo treatments which is the most horrible and dreadful part, I am doubtful of my strength to go through this ordeal.

Sifu I urgently seek your advise and response.

Name and country not mentioned

Answer

I am sorry and very surprised indeed that your cancer has reoccurred. This does not normally happen with students who, after surgery and chemotherapy, practice chi kung regularly.

At the physical level there are three possible reasons for your case. One, your regular chi kung practice is now clearing the root of your cancer.

For the past 15 months when you were diagnosed as free of cancer, what it meant was you were free from the symptoms of cancer, the root cause of cancer was still with you but was unable to cause any harm.

Now the root cause is being cleared out. Once that is done, you are really free from cancer. In the process of the root cause being cleared out, now symptoms manifest in the vagina. Earlier the symptoms manifested in the ovaries.

The second reason is similar to the first, except that in the first case it is your vital energy that is clearing the root cause, but in the second case it is the root case that is exerting itself.

In other words, in the first case your own regenerative power is stronger, but in the second case the root cause is stronger.

Three, you may be exposed to new factors that cause cancer, and despite your chi kung practice the new factors are strong enough to bring about a clinical illness. Some common cancer-causing factors are stress, severe grief or frustration, powerful radiation, and powerful electricity field nearby like a power station.

There are two more reasons at the metaphysical level.

Fourthly, it can be a case of karmic consequence. Something happened in your past, which includes your past lives, which is still imprinted in your mind or supra-consciousness without your normal conscious knowing. and it is now manifesting as cancer.

Fifthly, this is part of your developmental task. Whatever the possible cause, continuing to practice your chi kung will bring good result. Whenever you feel weak, discouraged or depressed, practicing chi kung will give you strength, hope and the will to live.

My personal opinion is that surgery will be fast and effective in removing the tumour, but I do not favor chemotherapy which will reduce your own resistance and life sustaining abilities.

The choice, of course, is yours; others, including the doctors and I myself can only make suggestions to the best of our understanding.

But there is one source that you must seek and can fully rely on, and that source is God.

Find a suitable, quiet place. Relax totally and get into a chi kung state of mind. Kneel down and say your prayers from your heart. Then repent for whatever sins you may have done in your past, which you may or may not know consciously. Ask Him to forgive you. Then you forgive someone whom you think has wronged you. Forgive him or her sincerely, and wish him or her well.

Next; bless someone sincerely. Then ask God to cure you, and ask Him to show you the way, which He will do in various subtle manners. If you pray sincerely, God always answers your prayers; this is a great cosmic truth.

You are such a lovely person. The least you deserve is to be healthy. God certainly will grant you that. I shall be leaving for Europe tomorrow, but do contact me whenever you have any question or need any help. You can e-mail me or call my mobile phone, and my phone company will contact me wherever I shall be.

If you have no objection, I would like to put the above in my question-answer series, as they may be helpful and inspiring to many other people. But if for any reasons (which you need not mention) you do not like the questions and answers to go public, I would accept your wish without any question.

Question

Your FAQ is amazing that I know something of what is real kungfu if I have a chance to learn.

But why Kungfu, Chi Kung and Taijiquan are not suitable for AIDS patients or HIV positive?

Could you tell me?

Guilherme, Canada (May 1999)

Answer

I have addressed the questions of AIDS and HIV before in my question-answer series, the latest being in Answer 12 of the April 1999 (Part 2) issue.

Firstly, please note I have never mentioned that chi kung, kungfu and taijiquan are not suitable for AIDS patients and those who are HIV positive.

In fact, I believe that chi kung will provide the best chance of overcoming AIDS.

But I mention that the intensive courses I offer are not suitable for AIDS patients and those with HIV positive. This is because I do not know enough of the effect of chi on the HIV (virus).

In particular I am not sure whether the chi resulting from my chi kung course might activate the HIV, thereby causing AIDS.

As I have always maintained that a good teacher must be both professional and responsible, I would not be practicing what I preach should I accept AIDS or HIV students.

Teaching something which I do not fully understand is being unprofessional, subjecting students to possible risk is being irresponsible.

The onus of professionalism and responsibility rests with the teacher, not with the students.

In other words, even if students with AIDS or HIV approach me saying, "Sifu, we know the risks and are willing to bear them", I would not accept them into my courses. It is like pupils telling their teacher, "Sir, we accept the risk of drowning, but please let us swim in the sea".

I also have a responsibility towards other students. Unlike in hospitals or special centers where safety measures are adequate, there are none in my courses. If an accident happens, such as during a self-manifested chi movement exercise an AIDS patient falling onto a healthy student and unwittingly stretching him, the former might pass on the HIV virus to the latter.

It is worthwhile to mention here that should any HIV patient think that since he (or she) is already afflicted with the disease, he would not care about the welfare of others, and join my courses under the pretense that he does not have AIDS or is not HIV positive he would be unwise and doing himself a great disservice. As I have said that I do not know the effect of chi on the HIV, the risk of him aggravating his problem is real.

Moreover, what is certain is that if his heart is malicious, he will not only deny himself the chance of a possible cure (which he may get somewhere else), but also deny himself of living his remaining life in a wholesome manner. If he can open his heart, despite his illness, he needs not be miserable. In fact the Chinese terms for being generous and being happy are "opening the chest" and "opening the heart" respectively.

Another legitimate question is "If I believe chi kung may turn out to be the best solution for AIDS patients and those who are HIV positives, then why don't I teach these people?"

The answer is as follows. I am a teacher, not a researcher. I know my limitations, so I leave the important job of researching into chi kung cure for AIDS for people who are better qualified than I am. I want to spend my time in areas where *I am sure* my effort will bring good results, not in areas where *I think* it may bring good results.

I am confident and competent when dealing with people suffering from diseases like cancer and cardiovascular disorders, as I know what I am doing and have good track records.

The need of these people is even more urgent than that of AIDS patients — the spread of incidence is wider, and the rate of death is higher and often quicker.

Cancer affects one out of five persons, and cardiovascular disorders is the top killer.

Question

I was wondering what would be the best way to balance chi kung exercises with cardiovascular type exercises.
Raymond, Ireland (October 1998)

Answer

I am not sure what do you meant by cardiovascular type exercises, but generally chi kung can be practiced by itself or in conjunction with other exercises. Chi kung is excellent for overcoming cardiovascular disorders. Many heart patients have recovered after practicing chi kung from me.

Qiqong for Health, Vitality and Longevity

To Me it is Almost a Miracle

18th July 1999

My daughter had an accident on April 21st, 1999. She was overrun by a truck. One of the back wheels rode over her buttocks. Three hours after the accident she was still conscious and was able to communicate with me. She went through multiple surgeries and the prognosis was uncertain.

I was worrying about the fixation of the fractures, but the nurses and doctors told me to wait and see if she could survive the first few days when it was very critical. I called Sifu Wong to help her.

He was in Toronto, Canada at that time and he was not able to come to Holland. He proposed to send chi from long distance. He did send the chi and said to me that he cleaned out the infection from the wound.

From then on the prognosis looked better, but you never know if that came from the surgery or the chi or both of them.

The most striking evidence I saw was when my daughter got severe abdominal/stomach pains several weeks after the accident when she was still in hospital. She threw up and had diarrhea for the whole night and the morning after.

When I came I immediately called Sifu Wong to overcome the condition. He was in Calgary, Canada at that time. I was worried my daughter would get dehydration. I came back to her room and held her hands. After about half an hour she fell asleep and from then on the pain was less and less.

Later on I asked Sifu when he did send the chi. (I did not tell him what had happened to my daughter.) He answered right away that he sent the chi immediately after I had called him.

The third time was when he visited my daughter and give chi right away. She felt dizzy when she received the chi, and the next day she felt she had one of the best days of her life, although she did not realize it was because of the chi she had received. From then on she progressed rapidly.

Now she does chi kung regularly every day. It has been almost three months since the accident occurred. She can now walk for approximately one hour without crutches.

My feeling about chi kung is that it does not work in a dramatic manner from one second to another second; but it works in a more subtle and consistent way that sometimes is difficult to appreciate.

To me it is almost a miracle. From this relatively short experience I can conclude that chi kung has some place both in health and medicine and that "long distance" chi kung is not a far-fetched story.

Hadi Sutedja, D.M.Sc.
Orthodontist.
Rotterdam, Holland

Sharing The Happiness Of My Class

Pere Sabata
Marketing Executive, Spain

Dear Sifu,

I decided to write this e-mail for different reasons, but the most important is to share with you my happiness about the results of my Shaolin Wahnam Chi Kung teaching.

A student (Manel, male, 33 years old), was allergic, and had difficulties breathing.

His office is on the 4th floor and he could not walk up the stairs, he had to take the lift. Everyday he has to take Ventolin, which is a medicine for asthma.

After 1 month practicing chi kung every day, his breathing was better and he only has to take the medicine 1 or 2 times a week.

Then he attended to your Tai Chi Chuan course. He continues his chi kung practice and now he does not take any medicine, his breathing is good, he walks up the stairs to the 4th floor, and he is very happy.

He will come to the summer course in Camponuevo. He asked me about his daughter. She is 7.5 years old, and she does not want to eat. She does not have any appetite and she is often ill. I answered that he should ask you in Camponuevo. The whole family will come.

Another student (Gemma, female, 35 years old), had stress and she could not sleep. She often takes tablets to sleep. After 1.5 months, she sleeps well, she does not need to take tablets and she says she dreams like she was 20.

The other students told me that they were more happy and enjoyed chi kung. One student (Imma, female) has decided to assist in the summer courses in Camponuevo.

One student from my first course (Jordi, male), who went to the intensive chi kung course in April in Barcelona and to the intensive Tai Chi Chuan course in June in Barcelona, asked me if he could teach "Lifting the Sky" to his mother because she was very nervous.

She takes a tablet in the morning for nervousness and a tablet at night for sleeping.

She cannot come to my class. I offered to go to their house to teach her, with one condition that if after a few weeks she is well, she should tell other people about the benefits of chi kung. Their house is 15 kilometers from my house.

I taught the exercise without mentioning breathing, only the form, because she was worried doing all, the form and the breathing. So I decided she did not have to do the breathing, only enjoy the form.

Another day I am going to teach her the breathing.

One week later, she told me that she does not take the tablets and she slept well. It is fantastic, she could not believe it! She is very happy. This is the 3rd week after I have taught her. She does chi kung every day.

I want to comment on what happened this Friday (14.July 2000). I went to take my son from my parents' house. (It is 25 kilometers far from my house). He spent a few days with my parents, my sister, her husband and their daughter. They have health problems.

My mother has rheumatism, cholesterol, and problems with her eyes. My father has rheumatism and my sister is always very nervous. They did not want to listen to me about the chi kung benefits, they said that they cannot spend a quarter hour a day practicing chi kung.

But this Friday they asked me about my chi kung teaching. I explained my students' benefits and they said that they would want to do it. I could not believe it!

I was very happy and I scheduled Sunday to teach them, with one condition — they have to come to your intensive course in October in Barcelona.

This Sunday (16 July 2000), I taught "Lifting the Sky" to my mother, my father and my sister. For my parents I did not teach the breathing because they were worried to do both form and breathing. But I will teach when I see that they can, but my sister could do all. They enjoyed it.

When I said to them, "Smile from your heart," my heart glowed with happiness because they wanted to learn and I could help them. It was wonderful. When I said "good bye", my mother kissed me like I kiss my son. I love them and they were very happy.

This Monday, (17.July.2000), I went to visit a customer. I talked with the owner of a cake factory. We are good friends. I saw that he had acupuncture needles in his ears. I explained about chi kung and its benefits. He was very interested because he has anxiety problems.

He cannot come to my classes because he travels a lot. He said that if I could teach him, he would pay me what I wanted. I was surprised. I said yes, but as I am a trainee-instructor, he has to come to your class in October. I wish to teach him "Lifting the Sky". If he comes to your course in Barcelona I shall teach him free.

What do you think, Sifu?

Another reason that I write is about my wife. Our relationship is better than before. She has accepted that I practice chi kung 2 times a day. She still has her health problems but she does not want to practice chi kung.

I do not force her. I followed your advice, "let the energy do". She is going to be interested in chi kung little by little.

This summer we are going to Segovia and she is happy because while I am attending the chi kung courses, she will remain in Segovia with one of her friends and she has planned to go shopping. She loves that and I am happy too that she is happy.

I want to comment too that this last week I had a stomach ache. The pain at first was little, but every day it slowly became worse. When I was 22 years old, I started to work and I was very nervous. After 4 or 5 months of having stomach ache I went to a doctor and he said that I had a stomach ulcer. I overcame it with homeopathic medicine.

Now I have the same feeling, but the conditions are very different. I thought about it. I practice chi kung every day, two times, morning and night, every day abdominal breathing two times, and 3 times a week I add the dynamic patterns and once a week I practice the self-manifested chi flow. I did the same procedure for 3 months and I felt very well.

So may be I need more cleansing old blockages. I have decided to change.

Every day even after the stomach ache has gone away, I am going to do the following: dynamic patterns — 1 fixed, "Plucking Stars", and the others changing — enjoying the chi flow, and 3 times per week, self manifested chi movement.

I started the last Tuesday. I did "Carrying the Moon" for the stomach ache to go away, and it helps. Now I feel better.

The pain in the stomach is like a pressure at the ribs under the lungs, and also at the back at about the same height. I feel a pressure too in the throat and in the ears.

It seems that I have a bubble of air in the stomach, and when I do chi kung it moves and the air goes away across the mouth and the anus but after one hour the pressure comes back.

I thought too whether I had done anything wrong in my practice. So, I have not done abdominal breathing even I usually feel good doing it.

Do you thing I am right?

Before June I did not have access to the internet. This is another reason that I send this e-mail. The company where I work gave me a portable personal computer and now I can log onto the internet.

So I could visit your web-site, and I found it very interesting. I follow the section on questions and answers, and I like it very much.

I do not want to forget before ending to say thank you a lot for all.

Really, thanks.

Pere Sabata
Email perecoll@inicia.es
20th July 2000

Editorial Note: This is a personal letter from Pere Sabata, a Shaolin Wahnam Chi Kung instructor in Spain, to Sifu Wong. It is published here in full with the sender's permission as it may be helpful to other people.

Question

For more than thirty years, you have been teaching Chi Kung.

How did you get in contact with this art and how did you begin to value it? What is the main contribution of this art on physical and psychical levels, and for long life?.

Could you please give some examples of illness cured by Chi-Kung?
Juan, Spain (April 1998)

Answer

I learnt the techniques from various teachers, especially from Sifu Lai Chin Wah and Sifu Ho Fatt Nam. I also developed some of the techniques myself, and I benefited a lot from reading good chi kung books.

I first valued these techniques when they produced practical results for many of my chi kung students. Virtually all chi kung books mention that practicing chi kung can overcome a wide range of diseases and provide good health.

At first I taught chi kung to my kungfu students who were already healthy, so there was no practical way to confirm whether what was written in the books about curing diseases was valid.

But when I taught chi kung to the public, and many people who has suffered for years from various diseases like high blood pressure, cancer, asthma, diabetes, rheumatism, peptic ulcers, depression, sexual inadequacy and nervousness, told me that their so-called incurable diseases were gone, I had concrete evidence for the effectiveness of chi kung, and was awakened to the inspiring idea that some diseases were considered incurable only if viewed from the conventional western medical perspective.

Personally I have helped many people to overcome their so-called incurable diseases suffered for many years, like cancer, asthma, diabetes, cardiovascular disorders, peptic ulcers, rheumatism, migraine, insomnia as well as depression and nervousness.

Chi kung is an excellent remedy for both physical and psychical disorders, and for promoting longevity.

I have a student who is an elderly man living in Madrid who suffered from prostrate cancer. He had tubes inserted into his bladder to help him ease his urination. After practicing chi kung from me for about six months, he was free from cancer and threw away the tubes. His friends said that he looked much younger.

A middle-age woman from Sevilla was told to have a surgical operation to correct her heart disorder.

After about three months of chi kung, her heart specialist told her that her condition had improved and the surgery could be delayed. She then flew to Lisboa, where I happened to be teaching at that time, to have further chi kung instructions.

When I next saw her a few months later, she told me that her heart disorder had been cured without having to undergo any surgery.

A young man from Alicante suffered from diabetes since childhood.

All doctors he had seen and many of his friends told him he had to bear his diabetes for life.

He was overjoyed when I told him diabetes could be overcome by practicing chi kung.

He told me I was the first person to tell him that diabetes can be cured.

He practiced my chi kung diligently and within a month he was cured! His was my record for the fastest recovery from diabetes. Usually it takes about eight months.

Chi kung is probably the best gift to the West from the Chinese civilization.

It helps to answer two urgent problems facing the West today, namely overcoming a wide range of chronic, degenerative diseases, and overcoming psychiatric problems, including intra-personal loneliness despite material affluence.

But it is important to learn chi kung from genuine masters, who are now hard to find in both the East and the West. It is not uncommon nowadays to find people starting to teach chi kung when they themselves have learnt it for only three months or even three weeks.

Then their students and in turn their students' students also teach chi kung. It is shamefully incredible!

These bogus instructors think that they can become masters themselves by imitating the exercises the genuine masters teach. It is like observing for a few days how a doctor treats patients, then starting to treat patients themselves.

If this unwholesome trend is not checked, the West will simply miss this wonderful gift of genuine chi kung.

Question

I am writing to inquire about the relationship between the practice of qigong and the treatment of Parkinson's disease.

What are the benefits and how does the practice complement the western allopathic course of treatment with dopamine and agonists?

Phyllis, USA (August 1998)

Answer

I am not familiar enough with the western allopathic course to comment on it, so I shall answer your question from the chi kung perspective. Practicing chi kung is effective in overcoming Parkinson's disease. There is no need to supplement chi kung practice with any other medication.

From the chi kung perspective, Parkinson's disease is due to interrupted energy flow along the nerves. In more familiar western terms, it means that the mental impulses a Parkinson's disease patient sends (unconsciously) to certain parts of his body for certain purposes (such as to hold a pencil) cannot effectively reach those parts. Hence the function of his bodily parts are impaired.

The forte of chi kung is to clear energy blockage and promote harmoniously energy flow. The great advantage is that one does not even need to know where the blockage is; it is the nature of chi to flow to where it is needed most. When blockage is cleared and energy flow enhanced, the illness will disappear as a matter of course.

But you need to practice genuine chi kung, not some gymnastics or dance that claims to be chi kung.

Question

I have read in your book "The Art of Chi Kung" that practicing Chi Kung can be very helpful for people with mental illness. However, I have also read in other articles that Chi Kung is not for the seriously mentally ill.

Can you explain how chi kung helps?
Kathy, British Columbia (May 1998)

Answer

Chi kung, being an art dealing with the training of energy and mind, is effective for overcoming psychiatric disorders.

Chi kung, nevertheless, is an umbrella term for numerous arts of energy training. There are hundreds of types of chi kung with varying level of attainment.

Some types of chi kung operate at a lower, physical level, which is not much more than some form of gentle physical exercise.

Others lead to mind expansion and spiritual fulfillment, irrespective of religion. Hence, those who practice and teach chi kung at the physical level will think that it is unsuitable for the mentally ill.

Unlike conventional western psychiatric treatment which generally deals with the symptoms of the illness, chi kung deals with the cause. Many psychiatrists and psychologists even deny the existence of the mind, regarding it as a function of the mechanical brain.

Chi kung masters, on the other hand, consider the mind and body as one integrated whole, and for convenience of study consider a person to be made up of three fundamental elements, namely mind, energy and form, which are actually interrelated.

If a person's form is weak, for example, it will also affect his energy and mind. In everyday terms, if you suffer from a physical illness, you would have less zest for work and play, and your intellectual as well as intuitive abilities will weaken.

Chi kung training nourishes all the three elements.

In other words, chi kung practitioners are not only physically healthy but also full of vitality and mental freshness.

Mind training plays an essential role in chi kung. A chi kung practitioner learns to relax, focus his mind and then let his mind expand.

Just as when the form is strong and the energy is full, physical illness and organic malfunction can be overcome, when the mind is made wholesome through chi kung practice, mental diseases — by whatever labels its many symptoms may be called — disappears as a matter of course.

This is so because good health — physical, energetic and mental — is our natural birth-right.

In other words, if our body (and mind), which for convenience is classified into form, energy and mind, but are in reality an integrated whole, is working the way it should by nature work, no illness will occur.

The forte of chi kung is to maintain and promote this natural working of the body and mind.

Question

Sifu, I have been being troubled by asthma since a child. I feel hard to breath and sometimes have chest pains after drinking cold water and sports activities. I took a lot of Chinese medicine when I was a child but it did not help much and now I am 19.

Sifu, is there still a chance for me to recover from asthma? I love playing soccer but I cannot play for long. I do love other sports too but I can only be a spectator. I was a kungfu student too but had to quit because I was out of breath and had chest pains each time I finish practicing.

Sifu, please give me some advise to overcome my asthma. I have been suffering asthma for years and I really felt happy when I heard about Sifu's

Qigong in curing diseases.
Tiong, Malaysia (July 1998)

Answer

Many, many people have recovered from asthma by practicing chi kung. But you must practice genuine chi kung, not just some gentle exercises that claims to be chi kung.

Today, as in the past, genuine chi kung is not easy to find.

The crucial point that differentiates chi kung from gentle exercise is that in chi kung the practitioner actively, consciously works on his vital energy.

In fact, the term chi kung literally means "energy work". And the most fundamental aspect of energy work is to be able to generate your internal energy flow.

Once you can do that, you may channel your energy flow to your lungs to clear away toxic waste in your air sacs, to increase your energy level for kungfu or soccer, and to do many other useful things.

You do all these things actively, consciously — otherwise what you practice cannot be called chi kung.

The factors that cause asthma in you and other asthma patients, are also present for all other people.

Why, then, you have asthma but they do not? The reason is that their body (and mind) systems can function to overcome these factors, often unconsciously, but you have lost this ability.

They did not have to practice chi kung to have this ability; this ability is natural — to them, to you and to everyone else.

It is as natural for us to overcome asthma, cancer, diabetes, depression, anxiety or any label we may give to the countless symptoms of our body's disease, as it is natural for us to breathe and eat.

This may sound amazing to many people, but it is a great, simple truth — often expressed in the saying "the doctor does the dressing, God does the healing". Ask any doctor, eastern or western trained, and if he sincerely searches his heart he will tell you the same thing.

Some doctors may tell you that asthma is "incurable". This does not contradict the truth that by nature we can overcome all diseases.

What they actually mean is that according to their knowledge and training, they do not know how to help you restore your natural ability to overcome asthma. This of course is no slight on them; there are other things that they can do extremely well.

Those trained in Chinese medical philosophy, including chi kung masters, look at diseases from a different perspective.

They are not worried over such details as what pollutants chock your lungs, which parts of your lungs are affected, and what antidotes to use, but they are concerned with the holistic task of restoring your natural ability to overcome asthma, or any disease for that matter.

It is too complicated to explain the details here. (If you are interested, please see my web-site on good health). The masters summarize all the details by saying that your health will be restored if you restore your yin-yang harmony, and this is done by restoring harmonious chi flow.

Chi kung is an excellent way to restore harmonious chi flow, which is the Chinese medical jargon of saying restoring your ability to overcome disease, an ability which you naturally have but temporarily lost.

You stand a very good chance of recovering your naturally ability to overcome asthma, or any disease. Many people have done so.

You are only 19; you owe yourself and your parents a duty to live healthily and well.

Seek a real chi kung master to practice chi kung, not just to overcome asthma but also to enrich your life and the lives of others.

Question

My mother and grandmother both suffer from rheumatism. They have tried numerous ways to relieve some of their pains, but none seem to work. I read on your web-page that you have helped people to cure this ailment.

Is this true? How do you do it?

I do not mean to question your methods or motives out of disrespect, just curious.

Matt, USA (May 1998)

Answer

There is no doubt that rheumatism can be overcome by practicing chi kung. Hundreds of people have done that.

But you must practice genuine chi kung, not just some gentle exercises that claims to be chi kung.

The crucial test of whether the exercise is chi kung is whether the practitioner can actively manage his or her energy flow.

Genuine chi kung masters are quite rare nowadays.

Rheumatism is the result of energy blockage in or between body cells.

Hence vital energy (which is more than just oxygen) cannot flow through, resulting in an inability to flush away toxic waste and to bring nutrients to the cells, and such a condition manifests as rheumatic pain.

Chi kung is an excellent way to clear the blockage.

Question

For the past two years my girlfriend has been very susceptible to coughs, colds, and flu.

She was repeatedly told by her doctor that her illness was stress related, yet considering that over the past year she has become more content, we both find this difficult to believe.

From what I have read in your web pages I get the impression that her illness may be due to a problem with her chi flow.

I would be very grateful for any advice you could offer on this matter.
Peter, UK (January 1999)

Answer

In Chinese medical thought, there is only one disease of the body, although there may be countless symptoms, and ultimately it is caused by blockage of chi flow.

The intermediate causes may be many, such as bacteria attack, stress or external injuries.

Chinese physicians are not concerned with the intermediate causes; they overcome the root cause.

In other words, once harmonious chi flow is restored, the disease disappears, irrespective of the intermediate causes.

Question

My mother had a stroke almost two weeks ago.

I have been unable to practice since then.

The stroke left her paralyzed on her entire left side, but she has regained some of her speech back.

She was not expected to survive — the doctors telling me she would be dead within a few days from the original attack.

Answer

The following program may be helpful.

Prepare a bundle of salt as follows. Heat some kitchen salt over a small fire, then wrap it up with a clean (preferably white) cloth into a bundle about the size of your fist.

Let your mother lie down, sit or be in any suitable, comfortable position.

Briskly kneed and massage your mother from her head down her body to her feet with your hands.

Test to see that the heated salt in the bundle is not too hot that it might hurt her. Then stroke your mother with the bundle of salt from her head down her body to her feet.

Gently visualize during the stroking that the heat from the salt opens blockages in your mother. Repeat about 20 to 50 times.

While letting your mother have a short rest, you move yourself away, preferably in some natural surrounding with trees or plants. Stand upright and relaxed. Take a few seconds to listen to your breathing, and feel that your "heart" which does the breathing is resonating with the whole cosmos.

Perform "Lifting the Sky" for about 10 to 20 times, following the breathing procedure I have described in "The Art of Chi Kung" or "Chi Kung for Health and Vitality".

As you breathe in gently feel, actually feel, good cosmic energy flowing into you (you do not have to worry from where the cosmic energy comes, or to which part of your body it flows).

As you breathe out visualize the good cosmic energy flowing to your palms and be focussed there.

Then, when you feel that your palms are charged with energy, "stroke" your mother with your palms from her head down her body to her feet. Your palms during the stroking should be about 3 to 5 inches above her skin.

In a meditative state of mind, visualize the good cosmic energy flowing from your palms into her, revitalizing her and generating her own energy flow.

Take a deep, gentle breath at the start of your stroking at her head, and gently breathe out during the stroking so that by the time you have reached her feet, you have breathed out about 80% of your breath, still with 20" at your abdomen (or where ever you normally locate your breath).

Take a gentle, deep breath and repeat the procedure about 10 to 20 times. Later, when you are more proficient you can increased to about 50 times per session.

Immediately after treating your mother, adjourn to some suitable place, preferably with trees and plants. Flick your hands as if you are flicking away water from them. As you flick your hands, gently visualize that any negative energy that might have back-flowed from your mother into you, is flicked away.

Then perform "Lifting the Sky" for about 20 to 30 times. For the first 10 or 20 times, visualize that any negative energy which might have back-flowed into you from your mother is cleansed out (you do not have to worry how) as you gently breathe out.

For the remaining 10 or 20 times, visualize that you are being replenished with good cosmic energy as you breathe in (again you do not have to worry how).

Perform the whole procedure about 5 or more times a day, preferably at or near sunrise and midnight, but avoid noon. If you perform this treatment daily for a few months, you may see miracles happening.

Question

I have recently been struck down with stress, worry, fear as my business was taking a bad turn. I deteriorated to a stage that I could not count the fingers on each hand.

The abdominal breathing has helped significantly. I have been practicing Chi Kung for 6 weeks (Lifting Sky, Carrying Moon, Nourishing Kidneys) and a couple of dao yin exercises.

Currently I have improved my health from pure relaxing, Abdominal Breathing and Chi Kung, and Tai Chi (beginner).

I do however come from a traditional background of doing GYM (Progressive resistance training for muscles and cardiovascular for heart and lungs). I had to stop this recently due a medical problem which allowed the stress and other bad things to take control.

I do Gym to keep fit and improve overall body strength/ toning to cope with day to day work loads (carrying heavy boxes etc.). I have not trained Gym for 3 months and am struggling with my general strength.

If I give up my regular Gym and do my Chi Kung and Tai Chi will I be able to keep my strength without having to pull muscles or injure myself when the time calls for extra muscle strength. I can understand if I have been training for 2 or 3 years with Tai Chi and Chi Kung I would have the strength.

Does Progressive resistance training conflict with Tai Chi or Chi Kung or should I do both. I am currently struggling with a very painful right hand side (it feels as if my whole right hand side of body is poisoned).

This only happens when I think of work or as I am doing now typing on the keyboard of a computer.

When relaxed and not thinking of business, my right hand side is fine.

Even when I try to practice Chi Kung (Lifting Sky or just breathing in the Wu Chi position I feel pain in the right hand side of my body (starting at shoulder level down to lower back).

This pain takes a lot of my concentration away from exercise and I cannot focus properly on training.
Derek, Botswana (July 1998)

Answer

If you practice chi kung or Taijiquan correctly, you can be very powerful without having to work in a gym or doing any physical exercises.

This may seem incredible to many people, especially those in the West who are used to the mistaken concept that if one wishes to be strong and fit, he (or she) has to strengthen himself by doing physical exercises like lifting weights and running.

From the Chinese martial art perspective, this is reversing cause and effect. The ability to do physical exercises well is the effect, not the cause, of being strong and fit.

What, then, is the cause for being strong and fit?

The answer is having energy and the ability to manage energy well. Chi kung is the art of energy training, and its forte is increasing energy level and managing energy flow. Taijiquan, if practiced correctly, is a complete set of chi kung itself.

While it is not necessary, but if you like to work in a gym, your having practiced chi kung will enable you to do gym work better.

Personally I think that progressive resistance training is not suitable for people with medical problems, especially problems concerning the heart, the lungs and the nerves.

Such training is stressful not only to the body but more significantly the mind. Chi kung training is superior; not only it improves energy level and energy management, it is relaxing both physically and mentally.

It is a mistake to think that you need to be tensed to be strong. Kungfu (including Taijiquan) masters are powerful and calm at the same time. Top athletes win their championships only when they can be relaxed during their peak performance.

Nevertheless, you have to practice real chi kung or real Taijiquan, which is not easy to find. For various reasons, what is taught publicly today as chi kung or Taijiquan is merely gymnastic or dance.

Question

At first I did my exercises all by myself, but after around a year my friends asked - what are you doing, you seem much healthier and younger nowadays.

So I told them, and they wanted to learn for themselves. So I translated the instructions and we started a group.
Marianne, Sweden (July 1998)

Answer

Congratulations. I am glad that you have made some progress.

Question

After a couple of years a woman asked me if I was interested in teaching Chi Kung to disabled people, who had suffered from different types of psycho-somatic diseases for years.

They all were what we call hopeless cases, so they had nothing to lose.

The leader of the group is a General Practitioner with orthopedics as specialty. She participated too, and all of the group members gained better health after they had practiced Chi Kung for some months.

Marianne, Sweden (July 1998)

Answer

This is wonderful.

Nevertheless, it is not advisable to teach chi kung unless you are properly trained because it is easy to cause insidious effects which you may not know.

But it appears you have done very well.

Question

Is it possible that we can generate our chi to, say, our shin or inner forearm and it solidifies like the example a woman who does not train hardening and building scar tissue on her shin or forearm yet can generate power or energy to that part of the body for an intended purpose?

Jack and Steve, USA (March 1998)

Answer

Certainly, this is one of the basic skills you will learn in my intensive course.

But you will have to practice for some time — a few months or a few years, depending on various factors like your intended purpose and your diligence in training — before the effect has become lasting for practical use, like breaking through an energy blockage inside your body or breaking a brick with your head.

Question

In your book you wrote that too much chi kung is also not good. How much is too much?

I practice Chi Kung twice a day; in the morning about 15 minutes and in the evening about 30 minutes but it depends on how long my "self-manifested movements" last.

Is this too much, Sifu? Sometimes I feel like I have a flu and pain all over my body.

Lanny, Holland (February 1998)

Answer

A good guideline is that you should feel fresh and energized after your practice. If you feel tired, it is a clear sign that you have practiced too much.

Between 15 to 30 minutes is suitable for most people on most occasions. But sometimes, depending on various factors, 15 minutes may be too much, whereas 30 minutes may not be enough. Use the guideline I mentioned above.

Sometimes when your chi is cleansing your toxins out, you may feel uncomfortable. But this will soon disappear. Let your chi movements move spontaneously, unless they become too vigorous, in which case you can slow down by giving a mental instruction.

Different persons, because of different needs and conditions, react differently.

Question

How do I stop my self-manifested movements when I am tired but the movements will not stop yet? It happened to me one night.

I was too tired to go on but my body still made vigorous movements and would not stop (I had thought of my dan tian and my feet).

At last I managed to stop the movements. Then I sat down.

While I was sitting I suddenly felt unwell and my head started circulating again.

A voice in me (I guess) told me to stand up.

So I stood up and the movements began very vigorously again.

After about 30 minutes it stopped at last.

After that I felt very light and very happy (I wish I can always feel the same).

Lanny, Holland (February 1998)

Answer

Just ask your movements to stop. It may be amazing to the uninitiated, but it is that simple if you are initiated and know how to go into the chi kung state of mind. This is one big advantage of learning from a master personally.

Your experience is a good example of what I mentioned about chi doing its best for you if you let it flow where ever it wants after you have generated its spontaneous movement.

You stopped the movement with your mind power, but later when you let go, it started moving again for your benefit.

Question

After practicing chi kung for about 2 months I feel my intuition is going to be stronger. Very often my intuition tells me something but I do not want to believe and I keep telling myself that this is just an illusion.

This makes me very confused too!

Lanny, Holland (February 1998)

Answer

There is no need to be confused. Have an open mind and let events prove whether you have acquired better intuition or are just having illusions.

But remember, as you have done, some "heaven secrets" have to be kept secrets. You may do others and yourself harm by letting "heaven secrets" out.

If you are in doubt whether to keep the secrets or tell somebody as it would help him or her, sincerely ask God. If you ask your guardian spirit, the guardian spirit must be of a very high spiritual level, such as a Bodhisattva.

If the guardian spirit is at your level, or sometimes even lower than your level, obviously asking him or her may not be very helpful.

Question

Kian keeps asking himself : "Am I doing the right thing?". Because this happened to him while he was practicing chi kung: He saw his upper and lower body split up.

While he was standing and practicing chi kung he saw his lower body not in one line with his upper body.

Lanny, Holland (February 1998)

Answer

This was a spiritual experience, and is not uncommon when we practice real chi kung, not just some gentle exercises that claim to be chi kung. Kian experienced he is more than his physical body.

A good way to tell whether he is doing the right thing is to evaluate whether he is getting what the art is supposed to give.

Many people practice chi kung and taijiquan and feel nice, but they are not doing the right thing because despite feeling nice, they never get the benefits that these arts are purported to give, such as enjoying harmonious energy flow and internal force.

Question

Very often when he is practicing chi kung he feels cold. He feels like a ghost is standing near him and that is frightening him.

So he keeps asking himself is this just an imagination? Or can you get this too when you are practicing chi kung.

Lanny, Holland (February 1998)

Answer

If he feels cold (actually refreshed) but do not feel uncomfortable, that is all right. But if he shivers and is uncomfortable, that is not correct.

In this case he should stop the practice, rest for a while, then practice Lifting the Sky or Self-Manifested Chi Movement for a short time.

When one improves his senses, he or she may be able to see spirits, but they are nothing to be afraid of.

When your chi is powerful, ghosts and lower spirits cannot harm you; your chi is like electricity to them. If you meet ghosts, you should actually pity them because they are lost.

You can help them by reciting some scriptures of your religion. For example, Christians can tell them some teachings from the Bible.

In Buddhist teaching, if you recite the Amitabha Sutra or the Ksitigarbha Bodhisattva Sutra, or part of the sutras, you can help the ghosts.

However, what Kian felt might just be his own imagination.

Question

Since I have done the exercises I feel that my character is changing. Before I was always tried and tried not to be angry with anyone. But now I can lose my temper easily.

For my work this may be good, because I can make clear what I want.

But when this happens to my family it makes me very sad, because I do not want to hurt the people I love. They have never thought that I am able to do this.

Mentally I am stronger now Sifu, but do I have to go through all of these to get my inner peace? I just want to be calm, to be able to understand people better and have peace with myself.

Lanny, Holland (February 1999)

Answer

Do not worry. All these problems will soon pass.

You are passing through a transitional developmental stage. Chi kung gives you courage, and this is one of its many manifestations.

It is not easy, and sometimes unpleasant, to do the right thing, such as upholding principles or telling the truth.

You are directly experiencing the benefits of chi kung developing confidence and courage. This development may cause conflict with those who have been habitually treating you as someone weak and undecided, and hence took you for granted in the past.

Inner peace comes in many ways, and often it comes after you have built up confidence and courage. Obviously someone who is unsure of himself (or herself) and is usually afraid, has little inner peace.

You will certainly acquire these good qualities of being calm, understanding and having inner peace. But before the calm there is often the storm; before understanding, the doubt; and before peace, the conflict.

Question

About my health, I feel well. But sometimes I can not breathe easily and have some problems with my eyes.

It is strange, though some people tell me that may be I have too much chi. I have never stopped doing the exercises.

My intuition tells me that I have to go through all of these to attain what I aim at.

Lanny, Holland (February 1999)

Answer

Chi is cleansing out your toxic waste. I told you about such discomforts before-hand.

Your intuition is right. It will be a great pity if you stop at this stage, as you are about to make a breakthrough.

Editorial Note: Lanny did have a breakthrough. Please read about her **feed-back** below which she sent to me about two months after asking me the questions stated above.

Question

I had a discussion with someone about "being happy". I said that I feel happy because I am healthy, I have a lot of friends, I have enough money to support my own living and most of all maybe because I belief in God.

That person did not believe me. He asked me how could I feel happy if there were a lot of people who are suffering. After the discussion, I began to read a book "The Art of Happiness" written by the Dalai Lama and an American psychiatrist.

The Dalai Lama mentioned that friends, health and having enough money are the basic for happiness. But "mind" is very important. If someone has inner peace he/she will feel happy.

After reading that I just realized that maybe that is also one of the reasons which makes me feel happy: I begin to get my inner peace through chi kung.

I think I never can thank you enough for all the things you have taught me. As Daniel and Kay Siang said, just by talking to you we also learn something from you!

Lanny, Holland (September 1999)

Answer

When I taught you chi kung I knew you would be happy.

Being happy is one of the most common feedback I have received from my students who have practiced chi kung earnestly.

At one level you were right in saying that your happiness came from being healthy, having a lot of friends and enough money to support yourself, and your belief in God.

At another level you were not quite right.

There are many people who are healthy, have friends and money, and believe in God, yet are not happy — they often envy their friends and blame God.

On the other hand, even if you had no friends and no money, you would still be happy.

From the chi kung perspective, the reason for your happiness is very simple — and profound! You are happy because you have opened your heart.

That is also why you do not need any medication for your heart now — although "heart" in chi kung context means more than just the physical organ. When energy blossoms from the heart, that person will be happy.

Why is this so?

It is so because it is the natural way of things — just as when he opens his eyes he sees, when he thinks of food his mouth waters, and when food enters his stomach he produces digestive juices to digest the food.

Chinese masters discovered this fact long ago.

Did you know that the Chinese term for being happy? It is "kai xin" (or "hoi sum" in Cantonese), which literally means "open heart".

This "opening of the heart" is similar to what the Dalai Lama says about the mind being the most important factor for happiness.

In Chinese, the term "xin" or "heart" often refers to what in English would be described as "mind". "Xin" also refers to spirit.

This is one main reason why chi kung is spiritual. In chi kung, we work not just on our body, but more importantly on our energy and spirit. Chi kung is a process of spiritual purification.

Hence, when your heart is opened, you become intrinsically happy and peaceful, irrespective of external conditions! This is what is meant by happiness comes from the heart.

This is also why the same external conditions — like friends, money and other people's suffering — can make some people happy but other people sad.

Your friend who said that one could not be happy if other people were suffering, would still be unhappy when the suffering had been eliminated if his heart remained close. If you are well trained in chi kung, your own happiness is unconditioned by others' doing.

You are happy with yourself and with the world although you know that there is still suffering.

This does not mean that you are selfish or sadistic, but it means that operating on the same principle but at a more immediate and down to earth level, even though you may be unable to buy a big house although you would like to, or your poor friends cannot live like millionaires, you are not going to brood over such shortcomings but make the best of what you can, and improve yourself and others within your capabilities.

The Dark Side of Chi Kung

Lanny
Secretary, Utrecht, Holland

Dear Sifu,

First of all I would like to thank you for answering my mail.

After two months of stormy weather and always cloudy I begin to see the sunshine in my life again. I begin to see the colors of the rainbow clearly again and realize that the combination of those colors make a rainbow beautiful! I am 100% okay now.

I am glad you have warned me about these uncomfortable feelings.

Knowing that all these could happen because of chi kung and that they were temporary made me go on with my chi kung exercises.

I hope you can use my story for your web-site.

Because my body was vulnerable for certain kind of diseases I joined a group for your chi kung training about 13 months ago. After this training I practiced chi kung everyday and felt very well. It seemed that I am cured of all the diseases I got before. For months I have not been ill.

Last year I took a personal class with you.

The reason was because I wanted more than just to be healthy. I also wanted to get what I was looking for (and am still looking for) in my life, i.e. inner peace and emotional balance.

I asked you to teach me some exercises to attain what I had aimed to get.

After two months practicing the chi kung exercises I felt something was wrong with me. I began to feel pain all over my body, got an eye problem, sometimes I could not breath easily, got the flu several times etc.

Suddenly I got all those diseases again which I had years ago.

Also I felt very uneasy and was very confused. I reacted more with my emotions and lost my temper easily which made me very sad.

I just wanted to make clear what I thought or what I wanted for other people. But my words made them confused and sad. My reaction shocked them sometimes. I lost my ability to think twice before saying something.

To feel uneasy, to be worried about something which you did not know what, trying not to discuss things with other people because you were afraid you would hurt them with your words again, to be sad and to be confused — all these made me ask myself what I was practicing chi kung for.

I supposed to be healthy, to get inner peace and emotional balance, but instead I got those uncomfortable feelings.

But I was glad that you had warned me about these things. Also the things you wrote in one of your books, something like this: practice, perseverance and being assured that your master's method is the best for you are what one needs to attain what one aims at in chi kung.

Those two things made me go on with my exercises. And I am glad I have done this because after two months at "the dark side of chi kung" I feel much better now and those bad feelings are gone. I begin to see life differently.

Before, the only thing I thought was just working and working again.

I have never taken the time to look around me and to see the beautiful things around me. I have never taken the time to look at people around me, to observe them and to listen more to their inner voice.

I just, like many other people I guess, went right to my destination, not noticing that I had walked through a beautiful garden.

When I look at people now, I feel like I look at them deeply: I see their positive side and also their negative side. I realize now that "the dark side of chi kung" has taught me something.

I am glad that I can be one of your students. We always can ask you when we are confused about chi kung. You always take the time to answer our questions. You make your students have the feeling that you also care about them.

Not many chi kung masters do this.

Lanny
Fri, 29 Jan 1999
E-mail: lannyutama@hotmail.com

Question

My son and my wife have experienced pain due to minor health problems and I tried to send them chi and they both reported feeling "heat" and relief from pain almost immediately.
Patrick, USA (November 1997)

Answer

I am glad that you could help your wife and son to relieve pain. This is one of the benefits we can get from practicing chi kung regularly.

You should, however, try not to transmit too much chi to others till you yourself feel depleted of chi.

How much is "too much" is subjective, but a good guideline is that if you feel tired after transmitting chi, then you have overdone it. In this case you should replenish yourself with chi.

Another important point to bear in mind is to take care that the negative energy of the patient does not back-flow to your chi-transmitting hand.

This can be done by withdrawing your hand fast after the transmission. You should also cleanse yourself of any negative chi which might have back-flown into your hands and arms.

Both the cleansing and replenishing can be achieved by performing "Lifting the Sky". After you have performed this pattern a few times, visualize or imagine negative energy flowing out of your arms through your fingers as you lower your arms.

After you have done this for a few times, think of good cosmic energy entering you and replenishing you as you raise your arms and breathe in.

During the standing meditation after the exercise, feel that you are both cleansed and replenished.

Question

Does sexual activity which leads to release of sperm depletes the internal energy of the body and is it harmful to mix sex and chi kung together?
Eric, Malaysia (August 1998)

Answer

Yes, sexual activity reduces the internal energy of the body.

After practicing chi kung for some time, you may find your chi accumulated at your abdominal dan tian (or energy field), and it may manifest as a little drum on your abdomen.

If you engage in excessive sex, you can actually see the drum becoming smaller or disappear altogether.

Hence, in the past many masters advised abstinence from sex, at least for the first hundred days of chi kung training.

However, values have changed through times, and our demand on as well as standard of chi kung aimed at are not as high as those in the past.

Personally, I feel that while chi kung is wonderful, wholesome sex, especially when one is married, is also important.

If a person totally abstains from sex, his chi kung attainment would be better, but this is not necessary because he can still get wonderful results at a lower chi kung attainment level.

Thus, I would advise my students to enjoy wholesome sex, but do not indulge in it.

The above explanation is particularly valid for men.

As women do not discharge sperm in the sex act, I am not sure whether sex would reduce their internal force.

On the other hand, I am quite sure that wholesome sex is beneficial to women — biologically as well as emotionally.

On a positive note, chi kung practice certainly enhances one's sexual performance and enjoyment — for both men and women. But we must maintain a good balance.

While sex is pleasurable, there are other things in life more important than sex. We should take the benefits from chi kung that relate to sex as a bonus.

If one practices chi kung just for sexual indulgence, then he or she is abusing a great art.

Question

You mentioned in one of your answers that Chi Kung SHOULD be practice after sex.
Dudley, UK (September 1998)

Answer

What I meant was that practicing certain types of chi kung after sex is advisable. I did not mean that one must (without fail) practice chi kung after sex.

Question

I have read many times that after normal intercourse during which a man ejaculates, he SHOULD NOT practice chi kung for a day.
Dudley, UK (September 1998)

Answer

This is a common advice from chi kung masters. It specially applies to hard chi kung.

Training hard chi kung (or martial art chi kung) where force is often exerted, after sex may drain the practitioner.

But leisurely practice gentle chi kung, like self-manifested chi movements, after sex can be beneficial.

Question

Should he only avoid certain kinds of chi kung?

For instance, should he avoid concentrating energy in his dan tian and instead perform energy gathering and regulating exercises like Lifting the Sky?

Dudley, UK (September 1998)

Answer

Yes, your observation is excellent.

Question

The primary justification I have read for discontinuing chi kung after normal intercourse in which a man ejaculates is that it can put too much strain your chi system.

Why do you suggest chi kung after sex?

Dudley, UK (September 1998)

Answer

Your justification is correct. There are many kinds of chi kung, as well as many different approaches even when practicing the same kinds.

While practicing hard chi kung after sex is generally harmful, it may not be so for a master.

I suggest chi kung after sex because it can replenish the energy lost during the sex. For a person who feels fatigue after sex, appropriate chi kung practice can revitalize him.

Question

How do I convert the aggressive/sexual energy into a form which is less disruptive and more healing?

Could the inflating/squeezing visualization be improved upon?

Are there any visualizations and/or other refinements that could improve my practice?

Josa, USA (May1998)

Answer

If you can learn this through an answer via an e-mail, there would be thousands of chi kung "masters" jostling in the street.

Do not continue this practice without proper supervision, if you do not want to head towards serious trouble.

There are many visualization exercises and other refinements, but they are not meant for someone like you who have not learnt chi kung properly.

Question

Can Chi Kung improve one's "LUCK" — making the right decision in business, investments, personal matters, being at the right place at the right time, meeting the right people, etc.?

If so, what kind or what technique?

Jo, USA (July 1998)

Answer

Yes, chi kung can improve one's luck!

Some people may find this incredible; they will be more surprised to know that in fact in the Chinese language the expression for having good luck is "good circulation of chi", which is "hao yun qi" in Mandarin pronunciation, or "hou wan hei" in Cantonese.

When one's chi is strong and harmonious, he is not only fit and healthy but also full of vitality, and has mental freshness and spiritual joy.

He will certainly be in a more favorable position than others who are sick, languid, dull and low spirited to make right decisions, and be at the right places at the right times.

How often, for instance, have you told someone who is sick, languid, dull and low spirited that he is lucky?

In Chinese philosophy, chi is the link between the physical (jing) and the spiritual (shen). When your chi is harmonious, your jing will be strong and your shen full.

In simple language, it means that if your energy is flowing properly, your body will be healthy and your intellectual and spiritual faculties will be enhanced.

It is not without reason that many eastern people believe that if your chi is circulating well, which is expressed as having good luck, even the devil is scared of you.

Any genuine chi kung exercise will enable you to have harmonious energy flow. Often it is not what you practice, but how you do so.

In other words, it is not so much the technique but the skill that counts. Even if you possess a wonderful technique but if you practice it as a dance or gymnastics, you will only get the benefits that a dance or gymnastics will give, such as elegant movement and muscular strength.

On the other hand, you can actually make any physical movements, or no physical movements at all, but so long as you practice chi kung, which literally means work on energy, you can achieve good chi circulation, or in Chinese "good luck".

If you can understand this, you will understand why I feel so concerned when someone starts teaching "chi kung" after having learnt it for less than three months, or when someone asks me to e-mail him a chi kung technique to cure his life-long health problem.

One of my senior students (who is a westerner) rightly commented, "it is simply amazing how little respect some people have for a great, ancient art. They think they can learn it enough by watching someone practicing it, then they teach it to other people."

Qiqong and Modern Medicine

Question
I am finishing my last doctorate courses in Clinical Psychology this year, and I am interested in conducting research in qigong as part of my dissertation.

In your opinion, what does the qigong field need in terms of research? Or, what would be worth studying?
John, USA (December 1998)

Answer
Congratulations on your completion of doctorate courses. You will find research into chi kung rewarding for yourself as well as other people, for there are many wonderful things chi kung can offer the modern world.

But I would like to modify your first question to "What do modern societies need in terms of research with special reference to qigong?"

This is probably what you meant.

The rephrasing of the questions will set the perspective right. I am sure the significance of this new perspective does not apply to you because you already know and value the contribution of qigong (chi kung), but it is important for those who think that when they do any research into qigong, they are doing qigong and qigong masters a great favor, when in reality it is the other way round.

Qigong and qigong masters do not need any research to confirm the effectiveness of qigong.

The real masters as well as those who have benefited from qigong know its effectiveness from their direct and personal experience. It is crucial for researchers to appreciate this point.

It will enable them to understand not only why many masters are not keen on research, but more importantly why those who jump on the chance of doing research with them may not be genuine masters, and consequently their research findings will not be valid.

Bogus masters who teach gymnastics or dance will grab the research opportunity to enhance their reputation.

The following true story may illustrate the attitude and perspective of many researchers.

One of my qigong students, who is a world renowned surgeon, knowing my successful work with many cancer patients, suggested to his colleague who heads the cancer department in their hospital to conduct some research with me into cancer cure.

The cancer expert — interestingly, she is publicly acknowledged to be a cancer expert although neither she knows about cancer (which is not a slight on her, as nobody knows what cancer is) nor is the recovery rate of her cancer patients high — suggested that I should submit a proposal and that I should pay for my expenses in the research.

My student asked why I should pay when actually I was helping her.

Her reply, which I believe would be legitimate from her perspective, was that the research would make me famous and I would subsequently earn a lot of money from the reputation I might gain from the research.

My student told her that I was already sufficiently known, that I already have a lot of students, and that I had no need for further publicity.

My stand was that if she was interested to research into my success with cancer patients, she should submit a proposal to me, instead of the other way round.

After all I would be sharing with her secrets which masters in the past might not even tell their daughters.

After rephrasing the question, let us now examine the answer.

Modern, especially western, societies face two urgent problems, namely degenerative diseases and spiritual loneliness. Chi kung happens to be excellent in overcoming these two problems. Chi kung has both sound theoretical explanation as well as adequate practical cases to substantiate this claim.

While overcoming degenerative diseases and overcoming spiritual loneliness through chi kung are both worth studying and researching into, I believe the first topic will be more appropriate at present.

You can take degenerative diseases collectively or take one degenerative disease individually at a time, such as cancer, cardiovascular disorder, diabetes and asthma.

Question

What is your concern or interest on how to integrate qigong and science?

Is there any point to this? (I realize the West has a rigid view, and needs to see 'hard' scientific data before implementations happen with medicine)

John, USA (December 1998)

Answer

The double standard wittingly or unwittingly adopted by many western professionals often baffles me.

In my opinion, there is hardly any "hard" scientific data on the success or even suitability of using chemotherapy, radiotherapy and surgery on cancer patients!

I sometimes wonder whether the professionals who administer chemotherapy, radiotherapy and surgery on cancer patients really know what they are doing.

Since they explicitly or implicitly admit they do not know what cancer is, and therefore do not know what it is they are supposed to cure, it is difficult for me to find their treatment objective, predictable or veritable — three crucial criteria for anything scientific.

On the other hand, qigong is objective (although it is often not quantified), predictable and veritable.

Unlike western professionals who are not sure what causes cancer, and therefore their recommended treatment is based on their subjective judgment, qigong masters are sure that illness, irrespective of the labels given to its countless symptoms, is caused by yin-yang disharmony, and therefore their treatment is based on the objective principle of restoring yin-yang harmony.

While western professionals cannot predict that chemotherapy, radiotherapy or surgery can remove the cause of cancer, qigong masters can predict that when yin-yang harmony is restored the illness will be overcome.

And while western professionals cannot verify whether a cancer patient is cured of his disease after he has undergone treatment of chemotherapy, radiotherapy and surgery (usually the patient has to wait for several years to find out whether his disease will relapse), chi kung masters can verify that once yin-yang harmony is restored, the patient is cured — and this is often substantiated by conventional medical tests.

The question of integrating qigong and science is irrelevant because qigong is already scientific. It is as irrelevant as asking how to integrate Chinese into a language.

Until and unless western medical scientists accept the fact that their way of looking at health and medical treatment is not the only correct way, there is no point attempting to integrate qigong with western medicine — just as until and unless western linguists accept the fact that western grammar and spelling are not the only ways to describe a language, there is no point debating whether Chinese is a language.

Say, you had diabetes. Your doctor told you that your diabetes could not be cured and you would have to take medication for life.

You practice qigong, and after some time you found that your diabetes had disappeared.

You see your doctor again, and he would say that you are just lucky or your case is a natural recession.

I would accept his opinion if your case is an isolated case, or even there are only two or three similar cases.

But if 40 out of 50 diabetics recover from their illness after practicing qigong, and the doctor still said it was luck or natural recession, I would consider him hopelessly closed to other medical thought and treatment.

If he challenged me to substantiate with hard data like sugar level and metabolism rate, I would not want to waste my time.

Meditation

Meditation Techniques for Achieving Outstanding Results
Richard Broadhead

Editorial Note: This letter was originally not written as comments, but as it may be helpful to others interested in mind training, the relevant part of the letter is reproduced here

Sifu,

You may remember that I have e-mailed you in the past, the last e-mail being just over a year ago.

You very graciously answered my questions, even providing me with a Taijiquan practice schedule and selecting two of my letters to be displayed on your web pages, for which I am honored and grateful.

Since my last correspondence I have completed my university degree achieving a first class honors, Bachelor of Arts in Linguistics.

This achievement was in no small part due to the focused and relaxed mind I achieved through daily sitting meditation, counting and following breath, during the months leading up to and during my final exams.

I have always been fairly relaxed about exams but these were the most important I have ever done and I found myself more relaxed than ever.

However the focused mind I obtained was an even greater asset and was something that I possibly lacked in the past.

I learnt the meditation techniques from your books The Art of Shaolin Kungfu and more recently The Complete Book of Zen and therefore have you to thank for the tremendous benefits.

(When I asked Richard for his approval to reproduce part of his letter, he was kind to provide the following invaluable information about his meditation for the readers' benefits.)

During meditation a few months before my final exams a thought arose. I was not thinking of my exams but concentrating on counting breaths but my subconscious was well aware of what lay before me.

The thought was as follows: I spend time reading and re-reading books and articles on my areas of study, as well as referring to lecture notes, and this still leaves gaps in my knowledge.

However, I need only read a novel or book of personal interest (such as one of Sifu Wong's) once and would be able to talk or write (if required) at great length and in great detail about such a book.

I dismissed the idea that this discrepancy is one purely of interest in the material, since I chose my area of study and it held my interest on a daily basis for three years.

I concluded that the difference lay in the way that my mind approached the different types of books.

I decided that the way that I would best learn was to aim to first understand notions and topics through reading without concern as to whether I knew specific terminology.

Therefore, for the next two months I meditated daily, counting and following breath, but for a brief period of each meditation I gently told my mind to focus on what I would be reading that day and to understand its content like I would any other book, that is, to read it like a novel, not a text book.

I cannot really say exactly how I told my mind to do this but I did. Then each day I was able to casually read relevant books and build up understanding. My studying seemed stress free and relaxed.

If I felt I was losing focus at any time I simply stopped reading and went for a breath of fresh air, a brief walk or picked up a book on an unrelated area and simply read at leisure for a few minutes. I needed only a few pages of brief notes for all of my studies.

When it came to the exams I found that I had no problems writing about topics and answering questions, important terms and words became like names in a story and I was able to achieve an excellent grade.

I am in no position to recommend that people copy my method of studying but I hope that my experience can exemplify to others how meditation methods taught by Sifu Wong can be used to find the best way for an individual to fulfill their potential in any area of life.

Richard Broadhead,
United Kingdom
E-mail: mailto:seniorlimpio@hotmail.com

Question

I began enhancing my studies by starting to meditate only a few months ago.

I have found it frustrating to initiate my meditation beyond a certain point where I began to feel that inner peace and calmness that I strive for.
Craig, UK (October 2000)

Answer

Meditation, which is called Zen in Shaolin nomenclature, is an essential part of genuine Shaolin Kungfu.

In fact I would go to the extent of saying that if there is no Zen in the training, it is suspect whether the kungfu being practiced is genuinely Shaolin. And Zen is found not at the highest level only, but right from the start.

Here I am referring to Zen or meditation in the true sense of the word, and not to the outward form of merely sitting cross-legged.

Hence, when a beginning student enters a heightened state of mind while practicing a basic Shaolin exercises like "Lifting the Sky" or Horse-Riding Stance, he is in Zen or meditation.

Obviously, to enter Zen one needs to learn from a master, or least from a competent instructor, and not just from a book or video.

If you practice Zen or meditation correctly and sufficiently, you will inevitably attain inner peace and spiritual joy.

This is a fact, and in principle is similar to saying if you eat correctly and sufficiently you will satisfy your hunger, or if you drink correctly and sufficiently you will satisfy your thirst.

Hence those who say they practice meditation but are still restless and confused, actually have not practiced meditation, or they have practiced meditation incorrectly or insufficiently.

Do not think that attaining inner peace and spiritual joy is a fantastic achievement available only in high level meditation. In fact such attainment is basic and occurs at the beginning of one's meditation training.

I am now (August, 2000) giving some Taijiquan and chi kung courses in Segovia, Spain, and presently just returned from completing a course on the "Fundamentals of Taijiquan".

In this course, where meditation was an integral part of the training, virtually every student felt peaceful and joyful after each session.

How do I know?

Many students explicitly said so, and one could also see the feeling of joy and peace on their face while they were performing the Wuji Stance.

Question

The results are spasmodic until I realized that it seemed to be my breathing that appeared to be incorrect.

I personally believe that this forms one of the corner stones of anyone's ability to practice martial arts and achieve results.

Craig, UK (October 2000)

Answer

Both your conclusions above are incorrect.

This is an example of the fact that many people, especially those learning on their own from books or videos, often draw wrong conclusions from their intellectual reasoning.

It is also an example showing that if one wishes to get good results from such arts like meditation or kungfu, he should learn from a master.

The fault in your meditation may or may not be due to incorrect breathing.

There are many meditation techniques, including those at the highest levels, where the meditator does not worry about his breathing and yet attains wonderful results.

If you are in doubt, some good advice is to forget about your breathing — just breathe naturally in your meditation.

Incorrect breathing in meditation is not a corner stone deterring good results in martial arts.

In the first place, many martial arts, including many kungfu styles, do not practice meditation formally.

Some examples are Choy-Li-Fatt Kungfu, Wing Chun Kungfu, Karate and Taekwondo.

Some exponents of these styles may say that they practice meditation, but in reality they seldom do. Yet the exponents can be formidable fighters.

Question

Can you advise on the best methods of breathe control to use in meditation?

Craig, UK (October 2000)

Answer

Different meditation methods will suit people of different abilities, conditions and needs. But the best methods naturally come from the greatest teachers of meditation, namely the Buddha and the great Bodhidharma.

Of the world's religions and spiritual disciplines, Buddhism is the one that pays the most emphasis on meditation, although many Buddhists themselves may not realize this fact.

There are, figuratively speaking, 48,000 meditation techniques in Buddhism!

The method most favored by the Buddha for most people is as follows.

Sit in a lotus or semi-lotus position. Half close your eyes and focus on the tip of your nose. Breathe naturally. Just be gently aware of your breath.

For example, if you take in a short breath, be aware that you take in a short breath. If you breathe in a long breath, be aware that you breathe in a long breath. That is all to it.

If you think the method is simple, you are perfectly right, but bear in mind that "simple" does not mean "easy".

All great teachings are simple — and profound. Only mediocre teachers and learners try to make simple things difficult.

Also bear in mind that this method is taught by the greatest of teachers, and if you practice it correctly and sufficiently you may achieve the greatest attainment any being can ever achieve, i.e. nirvana or enlightenment. But you, like most people, are not ready for such cultivation yet.

Nevertheless if you just practice correctly and sufficiently this simple method of being aware of your natural breathing, you will certainly attain inner peace and spiritual joy.

The method taught by Bodhidharma is also very simple.

Bodhidharma is the First Patriarch of Zen, which means meditation.

The method is as follows. Sit in a lotus or semi-lotus position. Do nothing and think of nothing. Dozen, the founder of Japanese Soto Zen, commented that if one can do just this, he is not cultivating to be Buddha, he is Buddha.

This method, which is the best for those who are ready, is not suitable for you and most people.

You will get better results by following the Buddha's method of being aware of your breathing. If you cannot sit in a lotus or semi-lotus position, sit upright in an ordinary chair.

Editorial Note: Craig promptly replied as follows.

Sifu,

Thank you for your response.

I have already begun using the information you have provided and I am finding that if I half close my eyes and focus on the tip of my nose and breathe naturally, as you said, it works.

Using this method, I am beginning to find that I can overcome the initial frustration of starting my meditation. It feels like there is a very gentle breeze blowing through my body.

It is wonderful!

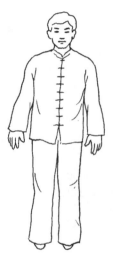

Standing Meditation

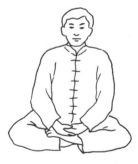

Single Lotus Meditation
(Buddha's Pose)

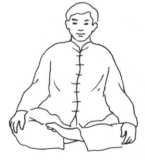

Double Lotus Meditation
(Lohan's Pose)

Question

I would like to know if you have heard of the meditation technique taught at the Monroe Institute, and how you would compare it to the chi kung you teach.

Is this meditation the same as what you would find in chi kung, or is it completely different?

Do you think chi kung would be more beneficial?

Ryan, USA (December 2000)

Answer

The meditation taught at the Monroe Institute and those taught in my chi kung courses are very different in both philosophy and practice.

Meditators at the Monroe Institute aim to examine various parts of their body and consciousness, whereas in my chi kung meditation we aim to have mental clarity and good health.

Our chi kung meditators also have a better awareness of our body and consciousness as the result of meditation, but these are extra bonus, not the actually objectives we set out to achieve.

The methods of these two systems are different.

Monroe meditators make extensive use of modern technology, like audio-visual aids, whereas we use none. Monroe meditators regard their teachers as guides, and generally treat them as peers, whereas we regard our teachers as masters and treat them with reverence.

Monroe meditation makes extensive use of visualization, during which the mind is free to roam. Monroe meditators are encouraged to have images, which are sometimes extraordinary.

For example, acting on cues from some audio-visual aids, a Monroe meditator may see in his (or her) mind a tree full of flowers, then the flowers turn into fairies, and he may find himself to be one of the fairies.

Basically we do the reserve in our meditation; we aim to remove thoughts and images from our mind.

If we use visualization, it is for a particular purpose.

For example, we may visualize chi or energy massaging our kidneys. Actually "visualize" is not a right word, but it is useful to give some idea to the uninitiated. To be more exact, we use our mind to direct chi to massage our kidneys, and we may or may not see this image of the massage.

We expand our mind, which is characteristically different from letting the mind roam.

When the mind roams, it encounters many images. When we expand the mind, we encounter the void.

Philosophically speaking, a roaming mind is phenomenal whereas an expanding mind is transcendental.

Of course I find the chi kung I practice more beneficial, otherwise I would have practiced Monroe meditation instead.

This is my opinion. Those who practice Monroe meditation may not agree.

Here are some of the many reasons for my opinion.

Monroe meditation works only on one level, that of the mind.

Chi kung works on all three levels — the physical, the energetic and the mind. Our results are holistic. We have a physically agile body, are full of energy, and attain mental freshness and clarity.

Monroe meditators do not aim for such attainments.

Even considering only the mind level, I regard my chi kung meditation more beneficial.

Monroe meditators let their mind dwells in images, which they apparently consider as real conditions of their consciousness.

We consider these images as not real, but are creation of the mind.

In our language, instead of letting the mind run wild, we tame the mind so that we may employ this most powerful tool for wholesome mundane application in our daily life, or for a glimpse of cosmic reality if we are ready.

In their visualization Monroe meditators have no control over their mind, but in our chi kung meditation we have full mental control. Like in the example above, after seeing himself as a fairy a Monroe meditator does not know what would happen next.

In our chi kung meditation we are sure of the effect.

If we use our mind to direct chi to massage the kidneys, chi will massage the kidneys; if we use our mind to send chi to the legs, chi will flow to the legs.

Question

Does Taiji or other martial arts enhance one's mental functioning?

In your book on Taiji you mention "mental freshness"; does this lead to enhanced intelligence?

Hua, USA (September 1998)

Answer

I often use the term "Taiji" or "Tai Chi" to refer to the external, dance-like movements of Taijiquan, and the term "Taijiquan" for the real art which focuses on energy and mind.

Taiji dance and external martial arts may enhance one's mental functioning minimally, but in many external martial arts sometimes a practitioner's mental functioning may be impaired through constant hits on his head that are routinely left unattended to.

But in great kungfu like Taijiquan and Shaolin, enhancing one's mental functioning is direct and purposeful.

Hence the result of mental enhancement in genuine Taijiquan and genuine Shaolin Kungfu is tremendous.

If you recall that training of mind is an essential dimension in Taijiquan and Shaolin Kungfu, you will better appreciate why a Taijiquan or Shaolin disciple will enhance his mental functioning.

There are many ways mind training is accomplished in Taijiquan and Shaolin Kungfu.

For example, in Taijiquan, every movement is directed by mind. In Shaolin Kungfu, a disciple is trained to focus his mind at a particular spot on his opponent so that a strike can "automatically" land there.

This explains why a dim mak master can accurately "dot" an opponent's vital spot even amidst much movement and even the spot is tiny. When the mind is trained, logically mental functioning is enhanced.

Yes, mental freshness leads to enhanced intelligence.

We are not particularly keen to know whether a "scientific" measurement or test of his intelligence quota will actually show an increase, but we know from practical experience that one whose mind has been trained through genuine Taijiquan or Shaolin Kungfu has better results than before his training in problem solving, academic studies, seeing relationship, understanding complicated information and other mental activities.

Question

I am 31 years old and have just finished learning the Dragon form and have started learning the Tiger form, both of which I am getting a great deal of pleasure out of learning & performing.

I have recently started meditation on a daily basis.

Gary, UK (December 1999)

Answer

Different masters have different approaches to practicing kungfu.

The approach I use is that after learning form, such as a kungfu set, you should spend more time practicing its combat application, instead of learning more kungfu sets.

Combat application has to be learnt and, more importantly, practiced systematically. Free sparring comes at the end, not the beginning, of this training process.

Meditation, which is mind training and not necessarily in the cross-legged sitting position, is practiced at all times, right from the very beginning of kungfu training.

Lotus-position meditation, which aims at the highest spiritual attainment, is attempted much later. A crucial component of my approach, which you seem to have missed, is force training.

Like meditation, force training has to be practiced at all times, starting at the very beginning.

There are many methods of meditation and force training — which are mind training and energy training.

In my school, the very first things a student learns and practices are "Lifting the Sky" and the Horse-Riding Stance, which are excellent methods for mind and energy training.

In "Lifting the Sky", among other benefits, the mind is trained to be one-pointed, and is then used to generate an internal energy flow or to tap cosmic energy.

In the Horse-Riding Stance, a student focuses his mind at his dan tian (or abdominal energy field), where he builds a ball of energy as the source of his internal force which he can use later.

The visible forms of "Lifting the Sky" and the Horse-Riding Stance can be learnt from a book, but the invisible skills of mind and energy training have to be acquired from a master.

Question

I have been practicing meditation for the past 3 years and I find that when I miss a few days I feel drained of most of my energy. Not just physically, but emotionally and mentally as well.
Matt, USA (January 1998)

Answer

Meditation is an advanced art. You should practice it when you are ready; in this way you would be able to get its best results.

You may practice it from scratch, but then you may practice wrongly and get adverse effect, or at best you will get little benefits even after practicing for a long time. This appear to be the case with you.

If you have practiced meditation correctly for three years, you should be healthy, peaceful and mentally fresh.

You should not feel drained of energy when you miss a few days of practice.

Question

In the last year I have spent a lot of time just thinking, seeking understanding, making questions and questioning the foundations of those questions.

I have spent time in an unschooled form of meditation, simply seeking to understand the basis of what is and what is not.

Ryan, USA (February 1999)

Answer

You would be interested to know that meditating and philosophizing are different. One may meditate on various questions, or one may philosophize on them.

The crucial difference is that in mediation, one uses his intuitive mind; in philosophizing he uses his intellectual mind.

It is best to learn meditation from a master.

If you do it on your own, even if you do not make mistakes, your progress will be slow and shallow.

Meditation is not just thinking about some questions, as the word may sometimes suggest in western culture, in which case it becomes philosophizing.

Meditation is the training of mind, and also the use of this trained mind to obtain wisdom.

Philosophizing is the training of intellect which usually involves reasoning, and also the use of this intellect to obtain knowledge.

When Plato said that the ideal form was a circle, this knowledge was obtained from philosophizing. He arrived at this conclusion based on intellectual reasoning.

When the Buddha said that the world we normally see is not ultimately real but is a creation of mind, this wisdom is obtained from meditation.

The Buddha's observation was based on his direct experience. He did not reason that the world is not ultimately real; he actually perceived this truth in his meditation.

Buddhism
and
Spiritual Cultivation

Zen Stories
Neil Burden, Canada

Dear Sifu,

I am glad to hear back from you.

I would like to relate a few stories I am working on after being inspired from your wonderful Book of Zen.

This first story I wrote down after you had asked me my progress in an e-mail:

A monk was practicing in a forest when he came across four pieces of wood.

The first he recognized so he ate it.

The second he had only heard of so he placed it in his tunic.

The third he had never seen so he threw it as far as he could.

The fourth he could not see so the monk ignored it.

The monk was practicing in the forest when he came across the four pieces of wood yet again. This time he used them for kindling that which warmed his very heart.

Who knew a piece of wood could be an empty mirror?

The second story, except for the last line, actually happened to me:

A teacher and his student were practicing in the forest when an old rotten tree came crashing down.

"Wouldn't it be ironic if the tree had killed us while we were practicing?' asked the student.

'It would be good fortune!' replied the teacher.

'How would it be good fortune, honorable teacher?'

'If a tree fell in the woods and no one was there to hear it would it make a sound?', retorted the teacher.

Just then a tree fell on him.

This last story was also inspired from real life.

It was the new year and Father gathered all his sons together.

'It is a new year, what plans do you have for the future, my sons?'

The third son spoke up first, "I will amass a store of gold and jade no one has ever seen father."

"I will build a pavilion in your honor, father" said the second son.

"I will rule the land with political savvy and diplomacy" replied the fourth son.

Everyone looked at the first son who said nothing, which was quite a surprise because usually you could not keep him quiet.

"What do you hope to do first son" repeated the father.

The first son smiled and proudly announced, "One day, I hope to have... a small wooden bowl!'

Thank you again sifu for your infinite inspiration.

Your humble student,

Neil Burden
Canada.
E-mail: neil.burden@hotmail.com
October 21st, 2000

Question

I have been studying Buddhism for a couple of years, mostly through books.

Jaber, USA (January 1999)

Answer

While books may provide useful information, Buddhism should be practiced, not just studied.

The best way to practice Buddhism is to follow the gist of Buddhism personally said by the Buddha, namely

1. Avoid all evil,
2. Do good,
3. Purify the mind.

Question

I find that Southern Ch'an is the school that fits my requirements the most.

I have found one group in Atlanta that practices Southern Ch'an, but I do not know Chinese and so do not know what is going on.

Jaber, USA (January 1999)

Answer

Practicing Southern Chan is a very good way to purify your mind.

Virtually all Zen masters have advocated doing away with language and pointing directly at mind.

Hence, not understanding the language of your Chan group is actually a blessing, not a hindrance, in your practice (not just study) of Chan.

"Doing away with language" implies that you should not verbalize or intellectualize what Zen masters have written or orally taught about Zen.

That is why when one goes into a seven-day retreat in Zen, he is not allowed to speak to anyone. That was why when students asked great Zen masters like Lin Ji (Rinzai) and Te Shan (Tokusan), the master shouted at them or struck them to keep them quiet.

"Pointing directly at mind" can be accomplished through sitting meditation where you do not think of anything.

If you imagine that you can achieve this in two days, or even two years, you are not ready for serious Zen cultivation. Just sit and meditate, and do not worry how long it will take you.

If someone lectures you on Zen in regular study groups, he is unlikely to be a Zen master; he may not even be a Zen practitioner.

At best he is a Zen scholar. But if you wish to study Zen so as to have some guidance in your Zen practice, read my book, "The Complete Book of Zen".

Question

I have tried many methods on my own but I now realize I need a teacher to guide me.

What should I do until I find a teacher?

Could you suggest a practice that may facilitate me until I find a teacher?
Jaber, USA (January 1999)

Answer

Do not just find a teacher, especially one who talks a lot about Zen. But find a competent teacher who shows you how to practice Zen.

Until you find one, just be keenly aware of your very present moment, no matter where you are and what you are doing.

Being keenly aware of the present moment is one of the best ways to practice Zen.

That was why when students asked great masters how to practice Zen, the masters said something like "Go and wash the dishes" and "When you serve me tea, I drink it."

Question

I am seeking very important information regarding myself entering monkhood in a Shaolin Temple in China.

I am earnestly looking for a very traditional, holy temple that maintains a low-profile, is secluded away from modern distractions.

I am very dedicated to the life of Buddhism/Taoism.

I would also like to supplement my training with chi kung. I want to study kungfu not as a combat sport but as a form of spiritual training, so I need a master competent in both of the disciplines.
Kevin, USA (July 1999)

Answer

Entering monkhood is an exceedingly noble but decisive decision; you have to consider very carefully.

If after very careful consideration, you are sure you want to become a monk, I would suggest that you fly to China (with sufficient money) and spend at least three months traveling all over the country to earnestly seek the master and temple you have in mind.

It is most likely that such a master and temple would be located in a very remote place, far from the noise of tourist centers and everyday civilization.

Read some good books on Buddhism. You may find my book, "The Complete Book of Zen" useful.

Meanwhile, practice even while you are still a lay person what a true monk would practice.

The three principal tenets of Buddhism are avoiding all evil, doing good and cultivating the mind.

The two pillars of Mahayana monkhood are compassion and wisdom.

Compassion can be readily realized through avoiding all evil and doing good, while wisdom realized through meditation.

Wisdom here is not just ordinary everyday wisdom, but cosmic wisdom, i.e. the understanding and hopefully the eventual realization of ultimate cosmic reality.

Question

Could you please tell me how archery refers to Zen?

Is it just a part of Zen, or does it belong to a total program?

Also could you recommend some good internet pages where I could read this. I am already archering, but just with the Olympic bow.

This does not satisfy me any more, because I would like to learn some more about the whole sport.

Treier, Switzerland (June 1999)

Answer

While Zen can be found in everything, there is no special relationship between Zen and archery.

We can employ Zen teachings and practice to improve archery, but archery is not an essential part of Zen — in the same way we can use weight-lifting to improve football or swimming, but football or swimming is not an essential part of weight-lifting.

Archery does not belong to a program of Zen training, but it may be used in Zen training if handled by a master who is well versed in both Zen and archery — in the same way as playing football or swimming does not belong to a training program of weight-lifting, but may be used to enhance performance in weight-lifting if the instructor is proficient in both.

Many people in the West relate archery to Zen, or relate motor-biking to Zen, because of the best-selling books, "Zen and the Art of Archery" and "The Zen of Motorcycle Maintenance".

I read these books many years ago, but I am not sure if I have remembered the titles correctly.

While these two books are enjoyable to read and actually provide some glimpses of Zen — personally I think they are better in providing glimpses of Zen than many Zen books written by Zen teachers who seem to make Zen more puzzling — paradoxically I think the authors did not understand Zen in the way Zen is meant to be by Zen masters.

It would, for example, not make much difference had the authors used titles like "Tao and the Art of Archery" or "The Kungfu of Motorcycle Maintenance".

If you wish to read my explanation of Zen on the internet, please refer to my web-pages like **FAQ on Zen** and **Buddhism, Zen and Spiritual Cultivation**.

You may increase your knowledge of archery by reading about it, but no matter how much you read you cannot be proficient in the art unless you practice and practice it.

This is one of the biggest mistakes of many students, especially in western societies — they read about their art but do not practice enough.

Question

I was practicing Zen meditation with a group of people.

For about 25 minutes we did sitting meditation, then for about 10 or 15 minutes we did walking meditation, and we finished up with about 20 minutes of sitting meditation.

During the last 20 minutes, I was meditating normally, focusing on my breathing, when all of a sudden, I felt my thoughts (which had been with me on and off) disappear, as though they were water in a sink whose drain had just been unplugged.

Very soon afterwards, I felt a powerful, warm sensation growing out of my lower abdomen, and my vision (we were meditating with half- closed eyes) swam slightly.

I felt completely aware of the room around me and the sounds around me, and for that moment all thought I had of the past or present were completely gone.

The warm sensation growing from my abdomen felt so strong and so good. I do not think that I have ever felt such a powerful physical pleasant feeling before.

Although it was a very warm feeling, I did not sweat, and my body did not move or sag; in fact, all of the aches and pains I had from sitting still seemed to melt away like sugar in water.

It probably lasted around a minute, and then it slowly subsided.

I was so shocked by what had just happened that I could not concentrate for the rest of the session, but just stared at the floor and wondered what had just happened.

Please tell me, Sifu Wong, is this a normal occurrence during Zen meditation?

Or is this a very strange aberration?

Sage, USA (January 2001)

Answer

Congratulations. Your experience was a splendid development in meditation, and if you carry on your training you would soon attain a "satori" or awakening.

A good piece of advice is that you should continue your training as you have normally done. Do not make any special effort to train more intensely or for longer time. Do not long for a similar experience to occur.

If it occurs again, just enjoy it; if it does not, it does not matter.

When the time is ripe you will have a "satori". Do not chase after the "satori", let it develop naturally.

Your method is an example of meditating on Zhao Zhou's "wu", or "mu" in Japanese, which means "nothing".

Zhao Zhou (Joshu in Japanese), who lived to 119 years in 18th and 19th century China, was one of the greatest Zen masters in history. A monk asked Zhao Zhou whether a dog had Buddha nature. Zhao Zhou answered with an emphatic "no".

This was in direct contradiction to a basic Buddhist teaching that every sentient being, including a dog, has Buddha nature. (In Christian terms, every being is a part of God.)

This seemingly irrational answer has become a famous "kung-an" ("koan" in Japanese).

Zen students of the Rinzai tradition use this famous Joshu's Mu koan for cultivation.

Zen students of the Soto school meditate on this Joshu's Mu. (Rinzai and Soto are the two main Zen traditions today.)

Working on Joshu's Mu — asking why a dog has no Buddha nature, or meditating on nothing — has help many Zen cultivators attain "satori".

One famous example was the great Japanese master Hakuin, the father of Japanese Rinzai Zen.

Interestingly, Hakuin's favorite method of cultivation was not asking koans, which is the main method in Rinzai Zen, but meditating on Joshu's Mu. He would go into sitting meditation and visualize that from his abdomen to his soles he was Joshu's Mu.

Then one day, in a flash of illumination, he experienced "satori".

"Satori" or "awakening" is inexplicable.

This does not mean we cannot describe it in words, but it means that no matter how accurately a master may describe it, those who do not have an experience of "satori" would not really understand the meaning although they may know the dictionary meaning of all the words in the description.

A classic analogy is a mango. Suppose you had never eaten a mango. No matter how accurately one may describe its taste, you would still not know what it tastes like.

Nevertheless, despite its imperfection, a description is often useful; at least it gives some idea of what "satori" is. When you attain a "satori", you are awakened to transcendental cosmic reality.

Reality is of two dimensions — phenomenal and transcendental.

What we normally experience is phenomenal reality. Right now I am sitting on a chair and typing on the keyboard of my computer. As I look out of a window, I can see some leaves swaying in a gentle breeze, hear some birds singing, and smell the gentle fragrance of vegetation and of life.

All these are phenomena, which means "appearances". Phenomena are not absolutely real.

They are real only in relation to a set of conditions, such as the ways my eyes, ears, nose, and other organs interpret data. Another sentient being, such as a bacterium or a fairy, would interpret the same data very differently. A bacterium or a fairy would not experience any chair, keyboard, breeze, singing or fragrance the way we humans experience these phenomena.

In other words, in the same space and at the same time, different beings experience phenomenal reality differently.

When we can "see" through, or break down, these conditions which limit or imprison ourselves, we experience transcendental reality.

Transcendental reality is of different levels.

When you said "The moon shines brightly over the floating world", you were experiencing and describing phenomenal reality.

When you have attained "satori", depending on your level of transcendentality, you may experience "the floating world shines brightly over the moon", or "there is no moon and there is no world, just the floating and the shine".

Question

I am reading your book on Zen, and it is excellent as I have come to expect from you.

However, I notice when I read the gong-ans that are supposed to be difficult and profound I understand them, but the ones that are professed to be less profound totally baffles me.

Several sutras you wrote in your book were described as "the essence of the teaching" with commentary saying if you can understand this you understand Zen/have had glimpses of cosmic reality.

I find myself understanding those from the humble experiences I have had with cosmic reality, but the gong-ans I find truly baffling are ones such as the "Go and wash your bowl!"

Why is this, master?

Daniel, USA (September 1999)

Answer

Simplicity and profundity are relative.

Telling a lie, for example, can be very simple to some people, but very difficult for others.

Standing upright and relaxed with eyes close is simple to most people, but can bring profound effects on others.

When the master asked his student to wash his bowl, he was demonstrating both the simplicity and profundity of Zen.

Zen cultivation can be found not only in chanting sutras and sitting meditation, but more significantly in our simple, daily tasks, including eating our food and washing dishes.

When a student is ready, in a moment of thoughtlessness while eating or washing dishes, a majestic glimpse of cosmic reality may flash onto him.

Question

Usually when I meditate, specifically zhan zhuang, I let my body totally relax into position, and let "my spiritual bud blossom".

I lose all awareness of my body, it just disappears (a strange sensation!), but strangest of all are the lights. A fantastic show plays itself upon my "eyelids".

I also feel joy when this occurs. I have had this experience for a year, and for a year of research I still cannot find any specific meaning for it. My only guess is either virtue or qi.

But tonight something different happened.

I saw eyes when my eyes were closed! It was most strange, I am still not sure if they were not just some sort of reflection of my eyes. The feelings I got from them were sort of an encouraging self knowledge and confirmation of infinity. But the most dramatic effect of all was when I opened my eyes again. They seem illuminated, like a row of very tiny stars are on the rims of my eyelids.

Every one of these phenomena I swear I have experienced, as odd as it my sound, though probably not to you, which is why I am writing about it to you.

Are these phenomena real, or some creation of my mind to entertain me somehow? And if they are real, what exactly do they mean?
Daniel, USA (September 1999)

Answer

Your experiences show that you have made some remarkable progress in your training.

Almost every consistent practitioner has experienced similar happenings as he (or she) progresses deeper in his Zen or chi kung practice.

The advice given by masters in the past in such situations was telling their students not to be tied to these happenings or to attach any meanings to them. Just continue the training diligently.

When the time is ripe you yourself will have the answers to the questions you asked above.

Question

I have read that martial arts were taught for peace of mind and mastery over the human condition, but that proficiency in any of these was not of high merit without other accomplishments in the Shaolin Monastery.

What would these other merits be? Is mastery over the mind, or samadhi, a characteristic point of Shaolin teaching?
Zachary, Australia (August 1999)

Answer

Shaolin Kungfu, strictly speaking, is a means to spiritual cultivation.

The two cardinal merits of the Shaolin teaching, which is based on Mahayana Buddhism, are compassion and wisdom.

Yes, mind training is a characteristic point in genuine Shaolin training.

The supreme aim of the Shaolin teaching, which is the same as all Buddhist teaching, is to attain no-mind, which is actually all mind. By no-mind it is meant that the cultivator has freed himself (or herself) from thoughts, which in a series of stages transform ultimate reality into the phenomenal world.

When no thoughts arise, the phenomenal world (which actually means the world of appearances) vanishes, and the mind returns to its original state, which is ultimate reality.

In Zen terms, this is seeing your original face.

In other cultures, the same attainment is described variously as return to God's Kingdom, attaining the Tao or unity with the Great Void.

Question

Shaolin was the name of the monastery visited by Bodhidhamma who first taught movements to the monks. This name, Shaolin, means 'young forest'.
Zachary, Australia (August 1999)

Answer

"Shao" literally means "young", and "lin" literally means "forest". But that was not how the famous monastery got its name.

According to the Shaolin tradition, when the great Indian monk, Batuo (not Bodhidharma) who built the monastery with imperial help requested Emperor Xiao Wen to name the monastery, the emperor said, "This monastery is on the Shao Shi mountain range (of Song Mountain), and these two cypress tress (still standing in front of the temple gate) form the Chinese character 'lin'; hence the monastery shall be called Shaolin."

Question

Was this first monastery Buddhist or Taoist or Confucian? Are these three interconnected?
Zachary, Australia (August 1999)

Answer

The monastery has been Buddhist since its first establishment till now.

But people of different religions, including Taoists, Confucians, Christians and Muslims, have studied in the Shaolin Monastery.

No, Buddhism, Taoism and Confucianism are not inter-connected; they are separate religions.

Nevertheless, one can be a good Buddhist, good Taoist, and good Confucian all at the same time.

In fact this is what most Chinese are!

Question

A Chinese Malaysian classmate has suggested that Taoist and Buddhist philosophies are irreconcilable.

I have read that the Chinese are renowned for the adaptation of new thought into old culture, and that Buddhism was readily absorbed within the existing belief systems of the time.

Could you clear up this dilemma?

Zachary, Australia (August 1999)

Answer

There is no dilemma if we view the situation from the Chinese perspective.

The apparent confusion arises when one views a Chinese situation from a western perspective. The Chinese concept of religion is different from that of the West.

Actually there is no such a thing as a religion in Chinese culture!

That is why when you ask Chinese what religion do they profess — apart from those who have been converted to Christianity and Islam, who would then normally conceptualize religion in the western sense — many of them will have difficulty answering you.

In the Chinese language, the word for religion is "jiao" which means "teaching".

In Chinese, Buddhism is "fo jiao", which is the teachings of Buddhas or Enlightened Ones; and Taoism is "dao jiao", which is the teachings of Tao or the Way.

There is nothing against any Chinese, or anybody for that matter, who follows the teachings of the Enlightened Ones to follow at the same time the teachings of the Way, or vice versa.

It is perfectly legitimate, for example, for a person to practice compassion and wisdom, which are the twin pillars of Mahayana Buddhism, and at the same time believe in yin-yang harmony and five elemental processes, which are principal teachings in Taoism.

Hence, in gratitude for the benefits he derives from these teachings, he may pay respect to both Bodhsattvas and Taoist gods.

In Chinese societies in and outside China, Taoist gods are often worshipped in Chinese Buddhist temples (which are usually Mahayana Buddhist), and Buddhas and Bodihsattvas worshipped in Taoist temples.

Your classmate who suggested that Taoist and Buddhist philosophies were irreconcilable, was viewing the topic from a restricted perspective.

If we compare the rituals, customs and practice of Taoism with those of Buddhism, especially Theravada Buddhism, we can find a lot of differences and may conclude that the two religions are irreconcilable as the rituals, customs and practice in Taoism are generally not found in Buddhism, and vice versa.

A Taoist priest, for example, would never wear a Theravadin saffron robe, and a Theravadin monk would never write magical talismans. But if we go beyond the external appearances, we shall find that attaining the Tao and attaining nirvana are actually two different ways of describing the same highest spiritual achievement.

Question

I felt the need to try the Standing Meditation exercise thought by you, but I did it lying down. I relaxed my body and went into a meditative state. I saw myself walking by what I thought was a tunnel. There at the end of the tunnel was a small bright light.

Curious, I decided to go in and see where the light originated. The light was so intense. There was this immense feeling of love, compassion and contentment.

Then I heard a voice say, "Now is the time to ask for something". I asked that my back injury be fixed. (It had been injured 20 years ago, causing me a lot of morning stiffness and pain). Then the voice said, "Now would be a good time to leave", and I obeyed.

At the same time something else happened. I started doing the Small Universe and it felt wonderful! The next night a thin, dry, black-like substance came forcefully out of my mouth. It lasted only a couple of minutes but the expulsion force was tremendous! The next morning my back was no longer stiff.

It was a miracle.

One day a huge person at work suddenly lunged at me. Surprised, my body immediately went into a type of "warding off" stance. I remember strangely feeling very calm and relaxed.

Then I heard a voice tell me, "Find his center core". But I did not understand and I guess the voice realized this because he said, "Lightly move your hands up ... higher ... higher ... there ... now move them closer together".

My hands continued to move to what seemed to be an ever increasing feeling of energy. Then the voice said, "there, right there". My opponent suddenly went onto his toes, arched like the letter "C" and started going backwards. He went about 3 feet until his momentum was stopped by a safety shower. Afterwards, I could see that he was really puzzled. So was I.

Sifu, after being in "The Light", my outlook toward my life and others has changed. The things that are "God given" are the true treasures in life. I appreciate this living world more and the people on it. My love for my family and friends has increased to limits that are too hard to explain. Some of the thoughts from your book on Zen seem to come from my own heart.

With this in mind, could you please tell me anything about this voice I have heard, this guiding spirit? Why should I be blessed by their attention? *Clyde, USA (October 2000)*

Answer

I do not know who this kind being is or why he (she or it) wishes to help you; but I can offer some possibilities.

One, this is a manifestation of your past good karma. Some time in your past lives, you cultivated to a high spiritual level and the experience was imprinted in your consciousness.

Performing the chi kung exercise correctly led you to a deep level of consciousness where your past experience surfaced to help you.

Two, that was actually another being outside you, and for some reasons, he (she or it) manifested in your deepened state of consciousness to help you.

Three, in you deepened state of consciousness you have touched the Universal Consciousness (often called "God" by some cultures), and the Universal Consciousness manifested as the voice to help you.

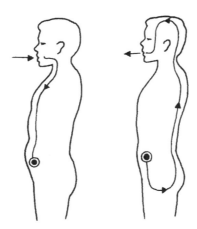

Chi Flow Direction in Small Universe

Question

After someone has experienced the Small Universe like I have, is it wise to try to do it again?

My energy flows well and my health has already greatly improved since doing it the first time.

Clyde, USA (October 2000)

Answer

Your experience of the Small Universe was the result of divine help or help from your deeper level of consciousness. Usually, but not always, once it has been generated in such a way, the Small Universe will go on naturally, sometimes you may not even be conscious of it.

Irrespective of whether it is going on naturally, it is unwise for you to meddle with it if you are ignorant of the required skills and techniques. If you wish to rekindle the Small Universe if it has stopped, or to enhance it if it is still going on, you should do so only with the supervision of a master.

But as you are already obtaining wonderful benefits from that experience, it is better to leave things as they are, and count your blessings. Should you want to do something, it is best to further increase your blessings by being charitable.

Charity is of three levels. The lowest level is the giving of material benefits, like monetary donation. The second level is the giving of service, like taking care of elderly people, especially your own parents if you are so blessed still to have them living with you. The highest level of charity is the giving of teaching, especially spiritual teachings.

One should give teachings only if he is qualified to do so. Giving false teachings, in whichever field, is not being charitable.

Question

I am new to the practice of Zen and am looking for some symbols to decorate my house with.

Christopher (June 1998)

Answer

There is no specific symbol for Zen, although many take the full and empty circle as a popular Zen symbol. It is full as it is a complete circle, and it is empty as there is nothing in it.

This symbolizes Zen, which is also full and empty at the same time, and can be manifested at different levels. The space in front of you, for example, is usually considered empty, yet it is really full of life — not only of microorganisms but also of infinite beings that we cannot see with our eyes as they have very limited capabilities.

To ordinary people, the phenomenal world is full of myriad entities, yet to the enlightened and the awakened it is empty — devoid of real substance as everything is merely a creation of mind. Indeed the word "phenomenal" means appearances.

The entities we ordinarily see are only appearances, and they appear differently to different beings, such as humans, bacteria and fairies, because of their different conditions.

Please refer to my web-pages on Zen for further information. You will have a more detailed explanation if you read my book "The Complete Book of Zen".

Question

Recently I have heard some pretty harsh statements being made against Zen Buddhism.

There are even books out that explain why Zen Buddhism and other philosophies and spiritual concepts are "wrong".

After reading your web page, I realize that many of these people writing these books may actually be practicing Zen Buddhism!

Realizing this, I feel that the writers of these books are being very hypocritical and judgmental. I want to stand up to them, but would that not be hypocritical of me (criticizing their religious beliefs)?

I realize that a Zen Buddhist should be tolerant of these "attacks" on Zen and Zen Buddhism, but I also feel that action is called for. I would very much like to know what you think.

Chris, USA (August 2000)

Answer

You are right in saying many people, including many pious Christians and people from other faiths, are Zen Buddhists without realizing it. They would consider it heretical if this idea is suggested to them.

Unlike in some other religions, in Zen Buddhism one needs not be exclusive and rigid in his beliefs and practice. He can believe and practice whatever he thinks is beneficial, and discard whatever is undesirable, without having to deny or contradict his own religious convictions.

One is hypocritical when his practice his contradictory to his beliefs. When you criticize another persons' belief, basing the strength of your criticism on your own beliefs, you may be critical or judgmental, but not hypocritical. But in Zen Buddhism we avoid both being hypocritical and being judgmental or critical.

This does not mean we do not stand up on our beliefs when attacked, but we do so calmly and sensibly.

When someone attacks our beliefs, our attitude is not of anger and aggression, but of pity and compassion. We are not angry and have no need to be aggressive because we honestly know that what we believe and practice are true and correct. Why are we so sure? Not through blind faith but by direct experience.

We know our beliefs and practice are true not because some authority tells us, but because we ourselves directly experience the truth.

This is the crucial point of the Buddha's teaching.

The Buddha advises us that we should not accept any teaching on faith alone, nor on the reputation of the masters, but examine and practice the teaching with an open mind, then accept or reject it according to our understanding and experience.

One becomes angry and aggressive only when criticisms reveals some flaws in his practice or affects his confidence in his beliefs. His anger and aggressiveness are mechanisms of defense. If their criticism really reveals our weakness, we thank them and re-examine our teachings to see if we have missed out something important.

But when we are so sure of our beliefs and practice, not through faith but through understanding and experience, others' criticism only reveals their shallowness and prejudice. We therefore pity them and feel compassion for them.

We share with them the wisdom that we are so blessed to have, but if they reject or debunk our sincere offer to help, we shall neither be offended nor disappointed, for it was never our intention to convert.

We respect the right and freedom of everyone to his beliefs and practice, and even if these conflict sharply with what we hold dear, we shall never despise or belittle them.

But we pray and hope that one day, as their karma improves, they too will have the wisdom and blessings that we are so lucky to have.

Question

I have read in various beliefs that sometimes an illness is a result of bad karma that has to be rectified, and that in some cases no one is allowed to interfere until the person has balanced his karma.

Is this a belief that you yourself subscribe to, and if so, is there any possible way of knowing whether or not a disease is your karmic fate?
Alan, Canada (May 2000)

Answer

To better understand your question about karma, it is helpful to remind ourselves of the limitation of words. This means the same words may have different meanings or connotations for different people, or for the same person in different situations.

In the widest sense, every event is due to karma.

Hence all illness, or good health, is due to karma. Here, karma means cause and effect, which actually is the original meaning of karma.

A person is ill now because of some causes in his past, such as being infected by bacteria two weeks ago, saddened by the loss of a friend, or born with a defective organ as a baby.

Each cause is also the effect of other past causes. For instance, he was infected by bacteria because he ate some contaminated food. The food was contaminated because the cook was careless.

The carelessness of the cook was due to his poor training, which was the effect of his low level education, which was in turn the effect of his parents being poor, and so on.

In a narrow sense, karma is frequently taken to mean the effect of some events in past lives.

This is the concept taken by most people, and is probably what you meant in your question. The division into "wide" and "narrow" sense of karma is arbitrary; the karmic process is a continuum.

In the example above, the cook's parents being poor was the effect of events in their past lives, and the cook being born into poor parents was also the effect of events in his past lives.

Now, suppose a person called P killed his friend F in a past life. He shot F's head point blank with a gun. The event was so vivid that it left a deep impression in P's mind, or soul.

Subsequently P died in his past life, and his body disintegrated, but his mind never dies. P, with the same mind, is reborn in his present body.

In his present life P has frequent and severe headaches. No doctors or therapists could heal him; it is due to his karmic effect.

But can his illness be healed? Yes. How? By rectifying or balancing his karma, to use your terms; or to compensate or to erase bad karma, to use other terms.

There are countless ways to rectify or erase bad karmic effects, and they can be generalized into two categories, namely to cultivate blessings and to cultivate wisdom.

Cultivating blessings is to do good, such as giving charity, performing service, and disseminating teaching.

Cultivating wisdom is to train the mind, especially in meditation, to perceive and experience reality at various levels, and ultimately at the highest, cosmic level.

Although both cultivating blessings and cultivating wisdom can be carried out at the same time, to most people cultivating blessings is preliminary: it leads to conditions suitable for him to cultivate wisdom.

If P habitually spends his time gambling and womanizing, lying and cheating, his habitual conditions are unsuitable for cultivating wisdom.

Even if he were to meet a great person who could help him to erase his bad karmic effects, he would not believe it and hence would not do it.

But if he starts to be charitable, to offer services to others, to seek great teachings, he is already on his way to cultivating wisdom. In proverbial terms, when he has accumulated enough blessings, his previous bad karma would be balanced or erased; when he is ready, the master will appear.

Depending on various factors, the overcoming of his illness, or the erasing of his bad karma may take many lifetimes, a few years, or an instant. And it can take many forms.

He may start to practice chi kung or meditation. As he progresses, he has glimpses of his past lives. Or he may meet a master who leads him back to his past lives.

Suddenly he sees, or re-lives, the event that causes his severe headache. He is in a battlefield. He and a few comrades were retreating under heavy fire. He sees F a few feet ahead, with his both legs blasted by a mine, and F is begging the running soldiers to kill him to end his agony. No one stops because the enemy is closing in. P hesitates a moment. Should he go over to help his friend but face the risk of being caught by the enemy. P goes over and tries to carry F on his shoulder.

"It's no use, mate!" F cries. "Kill me, kill me to end the agony," F pleads. P hesitates again. "Don't wait. Help me, please help me, shot my head." P places his gun at F's head and fires a shot.

This experience would balance or erase P's karmic effect, and he would be healed of his severe headache. He would also acquire some cosmic wisdom.

This example also shows that the question whether another person is allowed to interfere with another person's karma, is irrelevant. As in common in such cases whether the metaphysical is involved, there are no simple "yes" and "no" answers.

The answers depend on various factors, such as different interpretations of respective key words as well the spiritual understanding of the persons involved.

If an illness does not respond to medical treatments, and practicing chi kung for some time does not heal it, it is likely that the illness is due to karmic effect of a past life.

Performing an advanced self-manifested chi movement exercise to cleanse out deep rooted emotions can help.

A faster alternative is to lead the person to re-live his past life. Both types of chi kung exercises must be done by a master.

Some of my students had illness due to such karmic effect. Re-living past lives in self-manifested chi flow and in meditation proved to be very effective in overcoming their illness.

Question

I wondered if you were familiar with a Czech magician and mystic by the name of Franz Bardon, and his works, and what your opinions of his teachings were.
Alan, Canada (May 2000)

Answer

I am sorry I do not know about Franc Bardon or his works.

Nevertheless, the following information is very important to anyone studying or practicing magic. Magic is neither black nor white, or putting it in another way, it can be black or white, or somewhere in between. It is its application that makes magic white, black or gray.

Magic is real, and it involves mind over energy. It is utmost important for one who is blessed to have the skillful use of mind over energy, to use this ability always for good and never for evil. He may use it for his own good, but it must never harm others. This advice is for the sake and interest of the magician. If he were so foolish as to use his magic for evil, the effects will certainly bounce back on him.

An evil magician is punished not by God or Buddha or any Supreme Being, but by his own bad karma.

In other words, it is not that he is punished because he did something evil, but that he is punished as a result of his evil doing. The karmic law is universal and inevitable. Good cause brings good effect; bad cause brings bad effect — it is so simple, and so profound.

Whenever someone did something bad, the thought that preceded the bad action was already imprinted in his mind, and this bad imprint — like a negative in photography — will manifest itself according to its nature.

The manifestation may take different forms, but a bad imprint will always result in a bad effect. Hence, it is important for us not only to do good, but always to have good thoughts.

Question

I would like to know how to attain the state of no-mind? Is it through detachment, is it through functioning from a state of mind where one does not expect anything in return, meaning doing things for others without any expectation?

Or is it living for others without any expectation from others?
Anupama, India (March 2000)

Answer

No mind, or "wu-xin" in Chinese, is actually all mind.

It is a Zen term referring to a "state" where an adept has discarded his personal mind and attained the universal mind. This state of no mind may be attained at different levels.

At a lower level, an adept has a glimpse of cosmic reality. He may, for example, directly experiences that he does not have a physical body. In other words, he realizes through his own personal experience that the phenomenal world is unreal.

Should anyone think this is impossible or this merely exists in spiritual texts, let him be assured that some of my students have had such an experience. In Zen, this is called an awakening, or "satori".

At the highest level, an adept directly experiences that he is actually the eternal and the infinite! In other words, he attains nirvana, called by various peoples as return to God's Kingdom, merging with the Great Void or realizing the Tao.

Is attaining no-mind through detachment, through functioning from a state of mind where one does not expect anything in return, meaning doing things for others without any expectation, or living for others without any expectation from others? The answer is yes and no.

This is a good example illustrating that in the internal arts without deep understanding or better still personal experience, merely reading an instruction for a particular training may often give a misleading answer.

A master may rightly say that to attain no-mind, one must be detached. But you and most people's conceptualization of the master's statement is likely to be very different from what he actually means.

Detachment, not expecting anything in return, etc., are just prerequisites. They are needed for no-mind cultivation, but by merely being detached or not expecting anything, one cannot attain no-mind.

As an analogy, studying is a pre-requisite for passing an examination, but merely studying does not necessarily make you pass the examination.

Sitting in a lotus position or performing kungfu movements are prerequisites for meditation and kungfu respectively, but if you just sit in a lotus position or perform kungfu movements you are not performing meditation or kungfu.

The way to no-mind or all mind as taught by the Buddha consists of three stages, namely

1. Avoid all evils.
2. Do good.
3. Cultivate the mind.

One can attain the state of no-mind (but not its highest level) by merely cultivating the mind without avoiding all evils and doing good. But the result is certainly harmful.

This is not moralizing; it is a cosmic truth. If one develops a powerful mind without first purifying it, the power of an evil mind will first harm itself.

This explains why many western psychics, who did not have a spiritual base for their psychic development, had such miserable lives.

Mind training is very powerful and delicate. To cultivate for no-mind, Zen monks devote themselves full time and for many years in a monastery.

It is ridiculously egoistic for any person to imagine he (or she) can achieve similar results by practicing from a book for a few weeks — and then teach others.

It is also unwise to dabble in mind training without a master's guidance.

General

Question

What can be done for a master who has lost his way?

I will not mention his name as it might seem a lack of respect on my part, but he is a Shaolin grand master who seems intent on hurting people who love him, with lies and hurtful words, and gathering financial and public reward.

After what I have been through this past year I am ready to give up, but if there is anything I can do, I am willing. I am not putting my city down here because it might help identify him and I do not want him shamed in any way.

Sky, country withheld (February 1999)

Answer

The best thing that can happen to him to help him find back his way is to enable him to realize that Shaolin Kungfu is a means to spiritual cultivation. Not many masters, unfortunately, realize this.

I am here using the term "master" to refer to someone who is an expert in his art (as he interprets it), and in this case an expert in using Shaolin Kungfu for fighting.

It is of course legitimate to argue that this definition of a master may be invalid, because this "expert" does not have a complete understanding of his art.

It is pertinent to mention that my saying Shaolin Kungfu is a means to spiritual cultivation, is not a matter of opinion.

It is a historical fact that when Bodhidharma taught the Eighteen Lohan Hands which later developed into Shaolin Kungfu, his aim was to help the Shaolin monks in their spiritual cultivation.

It is also a historical fact that the greatest Shaolin masters were highly spiritual, and they attained their spirituality not through scripture studies but through kungfu training(which includes chi kung and Zen.

If one examines the philosophy of Shaolin Kungfu, he will find that the highest aim is spiritual, often concisely expressed in the Chinese phrase "xiu xin yang xing", which means "cultivating the heart to nourish the Buddha nature".

If he examines the practice of Shaolin Kungfu, he will find that the highest skill and technique is meditation, which is the essential path to the greatest spiritual attainment.

The most typical image of a great Shaolin master is not depicting him in a gruesome fight but depicting him in serene meditation.

A practical question is how would you help that master in this direction. Here are some suggestions.

Ask him politely, as a student would ask his master, whether it is true that Shaolin Kungfu is a means to spiritual cultivation.

If his answer is yes, ask him to elaborate. If his answer is no, tell him my views and ask him to comment. Whatever he says, do not argue with him.

Your purpose is not to show him how smart you are, but to tactfully expose him to the spiritual aspect of Shaolin Kungfu.

Another effective way is to give him as a present a book with information on Shaolin spirituality. Without being presumptuous, my book "The Complete Book of Zen" is a good choice.

Ask him whether he could explain the spiritual aspects to you.

One should also note that spiritual cultivation can, and should, be attempted at the level appropriate to the cultivator's developmental stage.

For the master you mentioned, he should forget for the time being such questions as who God or Buddha is, or how to go to heaven, but focus on seeking peace with himself and with others.

Finding peace is an intrinsic process; it comes from within. One effective way he can find peace is to remain at standing meditation for a few minutes each time after performing his external kungfu movements.

Question

More than anything I desire to live among the mountains in peace and relative solitude, studying and becoming more whole. I feel that I am trapped in a conundrum.

To worsen matters, living in such a small town there are no teachers for the arts I wish to learn, and no masters to induct me. I also find myself feeling very lonely.

Matthew, USA (February 1999)

Answer

Peace and happiness are free, and can be found anywhere — on mountain tops as well as in busy towns.

Even when you have a teacher, the main part of the cultivation has to be done by you yourself. Masters do not simply materialize from thin air; you have to seek them, and when you are ready you will find them.

Many people can be lonely in a crowd, while the contented find happiness in their solitude. Seek beauty and joy in your daily life and in simple kind deeds no matter where you are.

Question

Is there a way to satisfy this yearning which rests inside me?

Is there a way that I might live in peace and harmony, as I learn to sublimate this longing?

Matthew, USA (February 1999)

Answer

The yearning is often the necessary first step to serious cultivation. To live in peace and harmony is natural; war and disorder are unnatural.

There are many ways to peace and harmony, and different people because of different conditions will cultivate in different ways.

For me, and for many people, practicing the Shaolin arts is a wonderful way.

Question

I hope you will not find this question impertinent. Please ignore it if you find it unsuitable.

Did your Sifus charge you a lot for your training? Why do you charge such a large sum for training (US$ 1,000 for 4 days)?

Michael, Malaysia (August 1998)

Answer

The question is not impertinent.

In fact I like your question as it provides me an opportunity to explain my fees although I do not need to give any justification.

My sifus did not charge me a lot for my training. Uncle Righteousness taught me free of charge; Sifu Ho Fatt Nam charged me only a nominal fee.

If I have to pay, I would never have paid enough. This is not an exaggeration.

They taught me not just the best Shaolin Kungfu, chi kung and Zen, but how to lead a rewarding life for myself, my family and other people, according to the highest ideals in the Shaolin philosophy.

To put in a nutshell, I have learnt and practiced righteousness from Uncle Righteousness, and impeccable morality from Sifu Ho Fatt Nam.

Then, why do I charge others US$1000 for 4 days of intensive training?

My fees, depending on how you look at them, can be very expensive or very cheap.

Compared to some instructors who charge US$10 for as long as you want to practice, or even the more expensive ones who charge US$50 for three months, charging 1000 for four days is certainly very expensive.

If you have been looking for genuine kungfu or chi kung, and have expressed that you would give anything to learn it, and you learn it in four days what others, if they are lucky to have the opportunity to learn genuine kungfu or chi kung, take twenty years to acquire, paying US$1000 is very cheap.

For someone who has been suffering from asthma, diabetes, cardiovascular disorders, cancer or any other chronic degenerative diseases, which he knows conventional treatment gives him little chance of recovery, and for which medical tests merely to confirm the illness is present, will cost him (or his insurance company) thousands of dollars, paying US$1000 to learn an art in just four days, an art which according to statistics gives him at least 60% chance of recovery if he continues to practice it for a few months, is very cheap.

I just received a fax from Douglas, my most senior student in Europe.

The following quotation may cause you to think that my fees are very cheap! This is just one of my many successful cases.

"Dear Sifu,

I got a call yesterday from M.A., the young mother from Alicante whose baby suffered from narrow arteries from the heart to the lungs as well as leaky ventricles in her heart.

She was thrilled at the progress that the baby has made. The doctor could not believe how good the baby looked. Her next checkup is August 21. She asked me if you would be kind enough to send energy to the baby again to ensure that no surgery will be necessary."

Intending students would have the following three legitimate questions

1. How do I know the kungfu or chi kung I learn is genuine? After all every one who teaches, believes or says his art is genuine, if not the best.
2. How can I be sure that I can recover from my illness?
3. Can I learn it in four days? I thought kungfu or chi kung takes years to master.

The answers are as follows.

1. Find out from reliable, established sources what genuine kungfu or chi kung is, and compare what I teach with what you have found out. Also find out from those who have learnt from me before, whether they are satisfied with my teaching, and whether they get the results promised.

2. No one, including me or the best doctor, can guarantee that his patients will recover, because recovery depends on other factors besides treatment. But I can say that at least 60% (actually closer to 80%) of those who suffered from so-called incurable diseases, regain good health after learning and practicing chi kung from me.

   I would not provide names because I respect the privacy of my students, but those genuinely concerned should have no difficulty finding out for themselves if they take some trouble to ask around.

3. Yes, you can learn the necessary skills and techniques in four days. Some of the skills are quite fantastic, such as tapping cosmic energy, and channeling the energy down your body to clear energy blockage! Students do not have to pay me any fees if they are not satisfied that the course objectives, which are clearly set out, have been fulfilled. If someone thinks that he should have a longer time learning, he should know that I charge for efficiency and benefits acquired, not time spent. If I take four weeks to give him the same benefits which I can do in four days, I deserve a lower, not a higher, fee.

The intensive course is not meant to make you a master. Its purpose is to equip you with fundamental skills and techniques so that you can competently practice on your own after the course.

You need to practice for at least a few months before you can have lasting good results.

For example, after the course you will know how to generate your internal energy flow, but you have to practice this for a few months before your internal energy flow can effectively clear your energy blockage and restore your good health.

There are two good reasons, among others, why I charge a high fee.

It is a practical way to ensure that a great art is taught to deserving students, and it ensures that they value the art and will practice it.

In the past I used to teach some very good kungfu and chi kung to students for free. Because they did not pay for the training, they did not value it and stopped half-way. They each saved a thousand dollars but lost an invaluable art, and some lost the opportunity to recover from their so-called incurable disease.

A person with serious kidney problems went on a local newspaper to appeal for public donation to buy a dialysis machine. I offered to teach him free, and a reporter who knew of my good records in helping kidney patients recover, spoke to him.

He replied that it was too troublesome to practice chi kung.

Some time ago there was frequent public comment on the high cost of maintaining dialysis treatment for kidney patients (which actually does not overcome the kidney problem, but prevents the patients from dying).

I wrote to the secretary of a kidney patients' association and offered my services free of charge to any of his members who are interested. He did not even acknowledge my letter, but a few months later he said they were not interested.

Many people claim that they would sacrifice anything to learn a great art. But when it rains, they would not turn up for training.

This does not happen when students pay a high fee.

On the other hand, some people even think they are doing their teachers a service when they pay a small fee to learn. But if the fee is high, they value the art and subsequently derive good benefits from their practice.

It is not just that they want to get back their money's worth; rather it is often the other way round, i.e. they already value the art in the first place, as evident from their readiness to pay a high fee to learn.

The tenth Shaolin Law dictates that the Shaolin arts are to be taught only to deserving students. In the past a student stayed with and served the master for a few years, during which time the master observed and tested the student to see if he was deserving. Such a method of screening students is not feasible in today's world. Willingness to make sacrifice to an equivalent value of US$1000 is a modern, albeit poor, alternative.

Of course there are many other factors contributing to make a student deserving. Hence, it does not mean that anyone willing to pay US$1000 will be taught. But as a working guideline, I would consider that anyone who thinks my art is worth less than US$1000 to learn, does not deserve the teaching.

US$1000 is a comparatively small sum to pay for the benefits one gets in my intensive courses. Ask kungfu students in general how many of them have internal force and can effectively use their kungfu techniques for self-defense, or ask chi kung students how many of them can tap cosmic energy and generate internal energy flow. Less than 20% will answer positively, and they probably have taken many years to acquire these skills.

Yet, my students learn the skills in four days, and through daily practice for six months will attain a level these lucky 20% attain in 10 years.

But my best kungfu and chi kung are still taught to advanced students free. And deserving, beginning students who cannot afford to pay get free teaching from me.

Question

Could you please direct me in the right direction to get to facts on the original Shaolin history with Bodhidharma and the Shaolin monks in the Hau-naun province in the Sau-shaun mountains of Northern China over 3400 years ago

Ed, USA (February 1999)

Answer

The best place to get the facts is at the Shaolin Monastery itself where its long history has been recorded in its Monastery Histories and kept in the monastery library.

However, I am not sure whether these original Monastery Histories were destroyed in the last great fire set by a warlord attacking a rival warlord who took refuge in the monastery during the Kuomintang period about a hundred years ago.

This is the northern Shaolin Monastery situated at the Shaosi Range of the Song Mountain in Henan (pronounced like "Her-nan") Province. The northern Shaolin Monastery was rebuilt by the present Chinese government about 30 years ago.

There was another southern Shaolin Monastery situated at Quanzhow in Fujian Province. This southern Shaolin Monastery was built by a Ming emperor following the tradition of the northern Shaolin Monastery.

The southern Shaolin Monastery, which was much smaller than the northern counterpart, was razed to the ground by the Qing army about a hundred and fifty years ago.

My great-grandmaster (i.e. the master of my master's master), the Venerable Jiang Nan, was one of the few monks who escaped. He passed the Shaolin arts to Yang Fa Khun, who passed them to Ho Fatt Nam, who in turn passed them to me.

The present Chinese government has uncovered the site of this southern Shaolin Monastery, and has expressed the intention of rebuilding it.

The original Shaolin Monastery was built by a great Indian monk called Batuo under the imperial patronage of Emperor Xiao Wen Di at the beginning of the 5th century.

This was about 1500 years ago, not 3499 years ago as you mentioned. The Shaolin Monastery was initially a Buddhist temple for the promotion of Hinayana Buddhism.

About 150 years later in CE 527 the great Bodhidharma, a prince-turned-monk, came from India to teach Zen at the Shaolin Monastery. Since then the Shaolin Monastery has become the fountainhead of Zen Buddhism, which is a major school of Mahayana Buddhism.

Bodhidharma left behind as a legacy three great sets of exercises, namely Eighteen Lohan Hands, Sinew Metamorphosis and Marrow Cleansing.

Eighteen Lohan Hands became the forerunner of Shaolin Kungfu, and Sinew Metamorphosis the forerunner of Shaolin Chi Kung. There has been no record inside and outside of the Shaolin Monastery of how Bone Marrow Cleansing was practiced, but from indirect evidence I believe that it was similar to advanced self-manifested chi movement with emphasis on cleansing the nervous system.

"Bone Marrow" in Chinese medical terms is not just the bone marrow in Western terms, but figuratively refers to the nerves.

The great Bodhidharma is honored and worshipped as the First Patriarch of the Shaolin arts, as well as of Zen Buddhism.

Question

I am now 15 years old. Am I too old to start kungfu?.
Kim, Malaysia (March 2000)

Answer

No, you are certainly not too old to start kungfu.

My oldest kungfu student is Robert Trout of New York. He came all the way alone to Malaysia and started learning kungfu from me when he was 87.

This itself was an achievement — many people after 70 dare not even go out of their house. He is now 90 and still practices his kungfu everyday.

When I first met him he was 85. He had a serious heart problem then and could not even walk properly. He invited me to New York to teach him chi kung, which not only cured him of his heart problem but also strengthened him.

I am very proud of him. He is an inspiration to all of us.

Question

Besides that, does size really matter if you want to take up martial arts?
Kim, Malaysia (March 2000)

Answer

One can practice kungfu at any age (of course leaving aside babies). Different types of kungfu, however, are more suitable for certain age groups.

For example, children between the age of 5 and 12 should practice kungfu of the more external type with a lot of jumping and stretching. As their bodies are still growing, they should not engage in force training that demands body conditioning, such as punching sandbags or striking poles.

Young people between the age of 13 and 21 can engage in "harder" kungfu but they must take care not to deform their bodies, such as developing callused knuckles or crooked shins. Their young bodies and minds are also not ready for serious internal force training.

Those between 22 and 49 are ripe for any training, but career and family commitments may sometimes need considerations. Those between 50 and 70 may not be agile but can still be fast, and are better at training that demands patience and endurance. Elderly people beyond 70 are generally too slow for vigorous actions, but can be powerful with flowing chi movements.

In genuine kungfu, size matters — to the advantage of the person. A good master will consider a student's size in selecting the right type of kungfu for him (or her). If he is small sized, he will be suitable for fast movements and agile footwork.

When his opponent attacks, he will not block but move to the sides or back of the opponent and counter strike. If he is big sized, he will make full use of his weight and strong arms. When an opponent attacks, he blocks head-on, moves straight into the opponent and strikes — without having to bother with such intricacies as dodging the opponent and avoiding his force.

In most other martial arts, where the same techniques are used irrespective of the size of the exponent, size matters — to the disadvantage of the person. In judo, for example, despite what many judokas claim theoretically, if you are small sized, you will find it much harder to throw a big sized person. In taekwondo, if you are big sized you will find it more tiring to bounce about before moving in with a flying kick.

Question

I have never practiced kungfu before and will soon turn 32.

Do you think that because of my present age (I am in good physical condition, although somewhat weak) it will be impossible for me to reach a level of mastery close to yours?

Most masters seem to have started when they were still children or teenagers.
Alex, USA (October 2000)

Answer

If you have a good master and you are willing to train hard and regularly, you will not only reach my level but can surpass me.

While many masters started young, many others did not. For example, the second patriarch of Wing Choon Kungfu, Leong Phok Khow, started practicing kungfu only after his marriage to his wife, Yim Yin Choon.

An adult has many advantages over a child or a teenager. Not only he is stronger, his learning capacity and retaining power are also better. He is generally better disciplined and more persistent in pursuing set goals.

Question

I have great respect for the philosophy/aims of Shaolin Kungfu and would like to be able to help introduce others to its benefits.

But how could I ever do this if it is already too late for me to reasonably expect to become one day a master myself?
Alex, USA (October 2000)

Answer

It is significant to note that in the Shaolin teaching, no matter how beautiful or noble the philosophy may be, it is always geared towards practical results. Without practical results, the philosophy is merely hollow words.

Therefore, Shaolin disciples do not just talk about techniques and internal force, but actually fight well in combat. They do not just talk about energy fields and micro-cosmic flow, but are actually healthy and full of vitality. They do not just talk about the depth of Zen but actually experience spiritual joy.

If you ever want to attain a reasonably high level in any of the Shaolin arts, it is also important that you aim to be a good student first before ever thinking of becoming a master.

In other words, think of training for your own practical benefits instead of thinking of training to teach others.

This is a more meaningful approach.

When you are working for your own benefits rather than wishful thinking, it is less likely for you to give up when training becomes demanding, which it certainly will when one hopes to attain a reasonable high standard as a student.

Only when you have become a competent practitioner, you may start consider more demanding training to become a master.

Experience has shown me that ten out of ten who said that they wanted to learn the art to help others, did not even have the endurance for the most basic of training. They simply had no knowledge of or respect for how deep the art is. They were not willing to train as a good student for three years, but expect to be a master in three months.

Conclusion

My Search is Finally Over

Sifu,

My search is finally over! Thank you Sifu for the inner peace I have received from your intensive Shaolin Kungfu Course.

I have been a practitioner of martial arts ever since I was twelve, and started training from your excellent books in December of 1996, when I received your "The Compete Book of Tai Chi Chuan" as a gift.

Soon I was using the techniques contained in your books in the classroom and even my local teacher asked me who I was now training with!

I now have almost all your books, with your Zen book just recently ordered. My aims and objectives I set for taking your course were

1. To thank you personally for helping me overcome the little injuries I have received over the years from training in other martial arts. Even before meeting you, I was able to heal myself with the techniques contained in your books.

2. To thank you for the time saved from having the correct training methods and access to the knowledge of the ancient masters.

3. To make sure my interpretation of your training methods was correct and to rectify any mistakes.

4. To experience the romance of the classical kungfu knight, traveling to Shangrila to be accepted by Sifu.

I achieved all these objectives and much more than words can describe. I feel the cosmic joy of inner peace. Joy in the knowledge that my search is over.

Now I must practice!

Your humble student,

Neil J.H. Burden
May 30th, 2000
Gabriola Island B.C. Canada
E-mail: neil burden@hotmail.com

Question

Hello Sifu. I met you last year during the November qigong conference in San Francisco.

I attended your workshops, and during the last day of the conference, we had tea together in the hotel lounge.

I wanted to express my thanks, and to let you know that Shaolin Cosmos Chi Kung is amazing. I have not experienced another Chi Kung style or teacher with the same results as Shaolin Cosmos Chi Kung.

Thank You for this special gift.

John, USA (December 1998)

Answer

Thank you for your feed-back.

While your achievement is no surprise to me, it will serve as an inspiration to many people, especially those who, for various reasons, have not experienced any remarkable chi kung (qigong) effects although they may have practiced what they think is chi kung for many years.

The sharing of your experience confirms for them that what past masters mentioned about the effects of chi kung is true if one has the chance to practice genuine chi kung.

Question

I have thoroughly enjoyed your books, the Art of Shaolin Kungfu and Art of Chi Kung.

I enjoyed your case histories as I am also a Western Medical Doctor.

Ian, Singapore (October 1998)

Answer

I sincerely believe that chi kung has a lot to offer conventional western medicine. If you practice genuine chi kung, not just chi kung forms, and understand its philosophy, you may one day be instrumental in helping conventional western medicine overcome many of its present problems.

My web-page titled **Qigong, a cure for cancer and chronic, degenerative diseases?** may provide you with much food for thought.

Appendix

TEN SHAOLIN LAWS

The Ten Shaolin Laws are non-religious, and transcends all cultures and races, i.e. people of any culture and race would agree that they promote values that are worthy and desirable.

Laws, in the Shaolin tradition, are not meant to be punitive or restrictive, but as practical means to help followers achieve set aims and objectives; in this case to help them attain the best possible results in practicing Shaolin Kungfu for combat efficiency, joyful living, mind expansion, and spiritual fulfillment.

The Ten Shaolin Laws are not legally binding; one cannot be prosecuted in a court of law if he breaks these laws.

However it is morally binding. But they are not forced upon the follower; the follower accepts them because he chooses to, because he believes they are helpful to him in his physical, emotional, mental and spiritual cultivation.

If he breaks the laws, despite sufficient warnings, he may be asked to leave the Shaolin training, not as a punishment, but because the training is not suitable for him.

THE TEN SHAOLIN LAWS

I ..../ We Shaolin disciples in all sincerity pledge to uphold and practice the Ten Shaolin Laws.

1. Required to respect the master, honor the Moral Way and love fellow disciples as brothers and sisters.
2. Required to train the Shaolin arts diligently, and as a prerequisite, to be physically and mentally healthy.
3. Required to be filial to parents, be respectful to the elderly, and protective of the young.
4. Required to uphold righteousness, and to be both wise and courageous.
5. Forbidden to be ungrateful and unscrupulous, ignoring the Laws of man and Heaven.
6. Forbidden to rape, molest, do evil, steal, rob, abduct or cheat.
7. Forbidden to associate with wicked people; forbidden to do any sorts of wickedness.

8. Forbidden to abuse power, be it official or physical; forbidden to oppress the good and bully the kind.
9. Obliged to be humane, compassionate and spread love, and to realize everlasting peace and happiness for all people.
10. Obliged to be chivalrous and generous, to nurture talents and pass on the Shaolin arts to deserving disciples.

Qualities of a Good Master

Having a good master is definitely a tremendous blessing in kungfu, taijiquan and qigong training.

As mediocre instructors are so common nowadays — some even start to teach after having attended only a few weekend seminars — finding a great master is like finding a gem in a hay stack.

Here are some guidelines to help you find one.

An Example of What He Teaches

A good master must be a living example of what he teaches. A kungfu master must be able to defend himself, a taijiquan master must have some internal force, and a qigong master must exhibit radiant health, as these are the basic qualities these arts are meant to develop.

A master of kungfu, taijiquan or qigong does not enjoy the luxury of many coaches in modern sports like football and athletics who often cannot dribble a ball or run a race half as well as the students they teach.

There are also some kungfu, taijiquan or qigong instructors today who cannot perform half as well as their average students, but they are certainly not masters, although as a form of courtesy they may be addressed as such by their students or the general public.

Understanding Dimension and Depth

Besides being skillful, a good master should preferably be knowledgeable. He should have a sound understanding of the dimension and depth of the art he is teaching, and be able to answer basic questions his students may have concerning the what, why and how of their practice.

Without this knowledge, a master will be limited in helping his students to derive the greatest potential benefits in their training.

However, especially in the East, some masters may be very skillful but may not be knowledgeable. This is acceptable if we take the term 'master' to mean someone who has attained a very high level in his art, but who may not be a teacher.

The reverse is unacceptable, i.e. someone who is very knowledgeable but not skillful, a situation quite common in the West.

A person may have read a lot about kungfu, taijiquan or qigong, and have written a few books on it, but has little kungfu, taijiquan or qigong skills. We may call him a scholar but certainly not a master.

Systematic and Generous

The third quality of a master as a good teacher is that he must be both systematic and generous in his teaching. Someone who is very skillful and knowledgeable, but teaches haphazardly or withholds much of his advance art, is an expert or scholar but not a good master.

On the other hand, it is significant to note that a good master teaches according to the needs and attainment of his students. If his students have not attained the required standard, he would not teach them beyond their ability (although secretly he might long to), for doing so is usually not to the students' best interest.

In such a situation he may often be mistaken as withholding secrets.

Radiates Inspiration

The fourth quality, a quality that transforms a good master into a great master, is that he radiates inspiration. It is a joy to learn from a great master even though his training is tough.

He makes complicated concepts easy to understand, implicitly provides assurance that should anything goes wrong he is able and ready to rectify it, and spurs his students to do their best, even beyond the level that he himself has attained.

High Moral Values

The most important quality of a great master is that he teaches and exhibits in his daily living high moral values. Hence, the best world fighter who brutally wounds his opponents, or the best teacher of any art who does not practice what he preaches, cannot qualify to be called a great master.

A great master is tolerant, compassionate, courageous, righteous and shows a great love and respect for life. Great masters are understandably rare; they are more than worth their weight in gold.

Useful Addresses

MALAYSIA

Grandmaster Wong Kiew Kit,
81 Taman Intan B/5,
08000 Sungai Petani, Kedah, Malaysia.
Tel: (60-4) 422-2353
Fax: (60-4) 422-7812
E-mail: shaolin@pd.jaring.my
URL: http://shaolin-wahnam.tripod.com/
index.html

Master Ng Kowi Beng,
20, Lorong Murni 33,
Taman Desa Murni Sungai Dua,
13800 Butterworth, Pulau Pinang,
Malaysia.
Tel: (60-4) 356-3069
Fax: (60-4) 484-4617
E-mail : kowibeng@tm.net.my

Master Cheong Huat Seng,
22 Taman Mutiara,
08000 Sungai Petani, Kedah, Malaysia.
Tel: (60-4) 421-0634

Master Goh Kok Hin,
86 Jalan Sungai Emas,
08500 Kota Kuala Muda, Kedah,
Malaysia.
Tel: (60-4) 437-4301

Master Chim Chin Sin,
42 Taman Permai,
08100 Bedong, Kedah, Malaysia.
Tel: (60-4) 458-1729
Mobile Phone: (60) 012-552-6297

Master Morgan A/L Govindasamy,
3086 Lorong 21, Taman Ria,
08000 Sungai Petani, Kedah, Malaysia.
Tel: (60-4) 441-4198

Master Yong Peng Wah,
Shaolin Wahnam Chi Kung and Kung Fu,
181 Taman Kota Jaya,
34700 Simpang, Taiping, Perak, Malaysia.
Tel: (60-5) 847-1431

AUSTRALIA

Mr. George Howes,
33 Old Ferry Rd, Banora Point,
NSW 2486, Australia.
Tel: 00-61-7-55245751

AUSTRIA

Sylvester Lohninger,
Maitreya Institute,
Blättertal 9,
A-2770 Gutenstein.
Telephone: 0043-2634-7417
Fax: 0043-2634-74174
E-mail: sequoyah@nextra

BELGIUM

Dr. Daniel Widjaja,
Steenweg op Brussel 125,
1780 Wemmel, Belgium.
Tel: 00-32-2-4602977
Mobile Phone: 00-32-474-984739
Fax: 00-32-2-4602987
E-mails: dan widjaja@hotmail.com,
daniel.widjaja@worldonline.be

CANADA

Dr. Kay Lie,
E-mail: kayl@interlog.com

Mrs. Jean Lie,
Toronto, Ontario.
Telephone/Fax: (416) 979-0238
E-mail: kayl@interlog.com

Miss Emiko Hsuen,
67 Churchill Avenue, North York,
Ontario, M2N 1Y8, Canada.
Tel: 1-416-250-1812
Fax: 1 - 416- 221-5264
E-mail: emiko@attcanada.ca

Mr Neil Burden,
Vancouver, British Columbia.
Telephone/Fax: (250) 247-9968
E-mail: cosmicdragon108@hotmail.com

ENGLAND

Mr. Christopher Roy Leigh Jones,
9a Beach Street, Lytham, Lancashire,
FY8 5NS, United Kingdom.
Tel: 0044-1253-736278
E-mail: barbara.rawlinson@virgin.net

Mr. Dan Hartwright,
Rumpus Cottage, Church Place,
Pulborough, West Sussex RH20 1AF, UK.
Tel: 0044-7816-111007
E-mail: dhartWright@hotmail.com

GERMANY

Grandmaster Kai Uwe Jettkandt,
Ostendstr. 79,
60314 Frankfurt, Germany.
Tel: 49-69-90431678
E-mail: Kaijet@t-online.de

HOLLAND

Dr. Oetti Kwee Liang Hoo,
Tel: 31-10-5316416

IRELAND

Miss Joan Brown,
Mullin, Scatazlin, Castleisland, County,
Kerry, Ireland.
Tel: 353-66-7147545
Mobile Phone: 353-87-6668374
E-mail: djbrowne@gofree.indigo.ie

ITALY

Master Roberto Lamberti,
Hotel Punta Est Via Aurelia, 1
17024 Finale Ligure (SV), Italy.
Tel: ++39019600611
Mobile Phone: ++393393580663
E-mails: robertolamberti@libero.it

Master Attilio Podestà,
Via Aurelia 1,
17024 Finale Ligure (Savona), Italy.
Tel/Fax: +39 019 600 611
E-mail: attiliopodesta@libero.it
OR
Hotel Punta Est Via Aurelia 1,
17024 Finale Ligure (Savona), Italy.
E-mail: info@puntaest.com
Web-site: www.puntaest.com

Mr. Riccardo Puleo,
via don Gnocchi, 28,
20148 Milano, Italy.
Tel: 0039-02-4078250
E-mail: rpuleo@efficient-finance.com

LITHUANIA

Mr. Arunas Krisiunas,
Sauletekio al.53-9,
2040 Vilnius, Lithuania.
Tel: +3702-700-237
Mobile Phone: +370-9887353
E-mail: induva@iti.lt

PANAMA

Mr. Raúl A. López R.,
16, "B" st., Panama City,
Republic of Panama.
OR
P.O. Box 1433, Panama 9A-1433.
Tel: (507) 618-1836
E-mail: raullopez@cwpanama.net
   taiko@hotmail.com

PORTUGAL

Dr Riccardo Salvatore,
Tel: 351-218478713

SCOTLAND

Mr. Darryl Collett,
c/o 19A London Street, Edinburgh,
EH3 6LY, United Kingdom.
Mobile phone: 0790-454-7538
E-mail: CollDod@aol.com

SPAIN

Master Laura Fernández,
C/ Madre Antonia de París, 2 esc. izq. 4° A,
Madrid - 28027 – Spain.
Tel: 34-91-6386270

Javier Galve,
Tai Chi Chuan and Chi Kung Instructor
of the Shaolin Wahnam Institute
C/Guadarrama 3-2°A-28011-Madrid,
Spain.
Phone: 34-91-4640578
Mobile Phone: 34-656669790
E-mail: shaolin@inicia.es

Master Adalia Iglesias,
calle Cometa, n° 3, atico,
08002 Barcelona, Spain.
Tel: 0034-93-3104956
E-mail: adalia@xenoid.com

Master Román Garcia Lampaya,
71, Av. Antonio Machad,
Santa Cruz del Valle,
05411 Avila, Spain.
Tel: 34-920-386717, 34-915-360702
Mobile Phone : 34-656-612608
E-mail: romangarcia@wanadoo.es

Master José Díaz Marqués,
C/. del Teatro, 13
41927 Mairena del Aljarafe / Sevilla,
Spain.
Tel: + 34-954-183-917
Mobile Phone: 34-656-756214
Fax: + 34-955-609-354
E-mail: transpersonal@infotelmultimedia.es

Dr. Inaki Rivero Urdiain,
Aguirre Miramon, 6 – 4° dch.,
20002 San Sebastian, Spain.
Tel: + 34-943-360213
Mobile Phone: 34-656-756214
E-mail: psiconet@euskalnet.net
Web-site: www.euskalnet.net/psicosalud

Master Douglas Wiesenthal,
C/ Almirante Cadarso 26, P-14
46005 Valencia, Spain
Tel/Fax: +34 96-320-8433
E-mail: dwiesenthal@yahoo.com

Master Trini
Ms Trinidad Parreno,
E-mail: trinipar@wanadoo.es

SOUTH AFRICA

Grandmaster Leslie James Reed,
312 Garensville, 285 Beach Road, Sea
Point,
Cape Town, 8000 South Africa.
Tel/Fax: 0927-21-4391373
E-mail: itswasa@mweb.co.za

SWITZERLAND

Mr. Andrew Barnett,
Bildweg 34, 7250 Klosters,
Switzerland.
Tel/Fax: +41-81-422-5235
Mobile Phone: +41-79-610-3781
E-mail: andrew.barnett@bluewin.ch

USA

Mr. Anthony Korahais,
546 W147th Street, Apt. 2-DR,
New York, New York, 10031, USA.
Tel: 917-270-4310, 212-854-0201
E-mails: anthony@korahais.com,
anthony@arch.columbia.edu

Mr. Eugene Siterman,
299 Carroll St., Brooklyn,
New York,11231.
Tel: 718-8555785
E-mail: qipaco@hotmail.com

Index